KV-406-611

Contents

Executive summary and recommendations

Background

1   Hospital acquired infections are infections that are neither present nor incubating when a patient enters hospital. About nine per cent of inpatients have a hospital acquired infection at any one time, equivalent to at least 100,000 infections a year. Their effects vary from discomfort for the patient to prolonged or permanent disability and a small proportion of patient deaths each year are primarily attributable to hospital acquired infections.

2   The costs of treating hospital acquired infection, including extended length of stay, are difficult to measure with certainty, but may be as much as £1,000 million each year. Not all hospital acquired infection is preventable, since the very old, the very young, those undergoing invasive procedures and those with suppressed immune systems are particularly susceptible. However, in 1995 the Hospital Infection Working Group of the Department of Health (Department) and Public Health Laboratory Service believed that about 30 per cent of hospital acquired infections could be avoided by better application of existing knowledge and realistic infection control practices.

The top five ways hospital acquired infections can attack

Blood infections

After surgery

Urinary infections

Chest infections

Skin infections

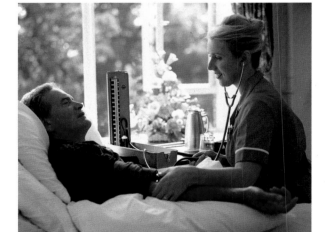

Six main things about hospital acquired infection

- Around one in 11 hospital patients at any one time has an infection caught in hospital.

- There are at least 100,000 hospital infections a year.

- They cost the NHS hundreds of millions £s a year.

- They can mean several extra days in hospital.

- The old and young are most likely to catch one.

- Hospital acquired infections may kill.

3 Against this background we investigated the strategic management of hospital acquired infection; what is known about the extent and cost of hospital acquired infection; and how well hospital acquired infections are controlled through prevention, detection and containment measures in Acute NHS Hospital Trusts in England (NHS Trusts). The main focus of the investigation was the work of the NHS Trust's infection control team, which has primary responsibility for, and reports to the Trust chief executive on, all aspects of surveillance, prevention and control of infection at Trust level. A key part of the methodology was a census of these Trusts.

Overall conclusions

4 During the course of our work we often saw the dedication of infection control nurses and doctors in preventing and minimising the problems of hospital acquired infection. We observed much good practice and real enthusiasm for it to be disseminated. But we are concerned about the remaining avoidable adverse effects of hospital acquired infections for patients' standard of care and health outcomes. And to the extent that some hospital acquired infection can be prevented, with our work suggesting the scope is significant, resources are tied up that could be used to benefit elsewhere in the NHS.

5 Good practice with respect to the prevention, control and management of hospital acquired infection needs to be more widely known and applied. Prioritisation of resources for dealing with hospital acquired infection is restricted by the lack of basic, comparable information about rates of hospital acquired infection. However, we welcome the work being carried out to develop evidence based guidelines, the Nosocomial *(hospital acquired)* Infection National Surveillance Scheme and the Department's new Clinical Governance and Controls Assurance initiative.

6 We believe that in many NHS Trusts there may be a growing mismatch between what is expected of infection control teams in controlling hospital infection and the staffing and other resources allocated to them. Hospital acquired infection is very costly and, to the extent that some of it is preventable, it is possible to improve patient care and save money. But it will be important for NHS Trusts to justify existing and additional expenditure on infection control against other uses of health resources.

7 There are many ways to build upon the work already carried out by infection control teams and others. It is encouraging that the Department has recently taken a number of initiatives to raise the profile of hospital acquired infection and improve its prevention and control. We urge that our recommendations for improving management and control of hospital acquired infection be considered quickly in the interests of better patient outcomes and releasing resources for alternative NHS uses.

Main conclusions and recommendations

Strategic management of hospital acquired infection

8 A number of NHS Trusts have put infection control high on their agenda, but health authorities and NHS Trusts generally could do more to improve its strategic management. A quarter of service agreements between NHS Trusts and their health authorities did not cover the provision of infection control services. Where infection control was covered, it was sometimes without input from the personnel with detailed knowledge about infection control, namely the Trust's infection control team and the health authority's Consultant in Communicable Disease Control.

9 The requirements within service agreements also tended to be in very general terms. For example, while 66 per cent specified the need to undertake surveillance to collect data on infections, only 27 per cent included the need to calculate infection rates. Lack of detailed specification within service agreements and lack of compliance with them means that many health authorities do not have all the data they need to assess NHS Trusts' performance in improving infection control.

10 In 1995, the Department issued guidance that gave NHS Trust chief executives overall responsibility for ensuring the provision of effective infection control arrangements. We found in the majority of NHS Trusts that direct chief executive involvement was very low. Few chief executives were members of their Hospital Infection Control Committee, the key management forum for infection control in NHS Trusts, and in 30 per cent of NHS Trusts neither the chief executive nor a nominated representative was a member. Fifty eight per cent of NHS Trust chief executives never received reports on resources spent on hospital acquired infection and less than half received reports on rates or numbers of hospital acquired infections. This suggests that in a number of NHS Trusts, chief executives may be unaware of the extent and cost of hospital acquired infection and how it is being addressed in their NHS Trust, though these aspects may be delegated to other senior managers.

11   Seventy nine per cent of NHS Trusts had an infection control programme, which generally complied with the Department's guidance on content, although in some NHS Trusts there were notable omissions in relation to the measurement of effectiveness, such as standards setting and audit. In the fifth of NHS Trusts that did not have an infection control programme, infection control was largely reactive in nature. Contrary to Departmental guidance that all chief executives should approve the infection control programme, only 11 per cent formally approved the programme. This may reduce the programme's authority within many NHS Trusts.

12   The Department's guidance states that there are advantages for the planning and implementation of an effective infection control programme if infection control teams have separate budgets. Only some 40 per cent of NHS Trusts had a separate budget for hospital infection control. Often these budgets do not include all the elements suggested in Departmental guidance and the amounts allocated to the budget vary widely. Most infection control teams considered that there had been little real term change in the amount of money spent on infection control in the last three years yet, during this time, expectations particularly in relation to a number of resource intensive activities have increased.

13   There are no Departmental guidelines on infection control staffing. Few NHS Trusts met the guidelines recommended by the Royal College of Pathologists on the amount of time that infection control doctors should spend on infection control.There are also wide variations in the ratio of infection control nurses to beds and, in some NHS Trusts, we consider that the number of beds that a single infection control nurse is expected to cover is unacceptably high. We are concerned that the wide variation in infection control team resources may represent unacceptable differences that could impact on the quality of care that patients can expect regarding hospital acquired infection and infection control generally in hospitals.

14   Over 60 per cent of infection control teams considered that they had inadequate clerical support, with 27 per cent having none. Lack of computer software and hardware was also cited as a major constraint in providing effective infection control. The Department's NHS Information for Health Strategy, which includes installing electronic patient record systems and reporting results of prescribing, should help improve matters, but infection control teams will need appropriate access.

Surveillance and the extent and cost of hospital acquired infection

15   The Hospital Infection Working Group believed in 1995 that it might have been possible to achieve a 30 per cent reduction in hospital acquired infection. Infection control teams in our census believed on average that a reduction of 15 per cent was possible.

16   Attributing costs to hospital acquired infection is complex and uncertain. However, a comprehensive study commissioned by the Department and undertaken by the London School of Hygiene and Tropical Medicine and the Central Public Health Laboratory suggests that hospital acquired infection may be costing the NHS as much as £1 billion a year. This estimate is based on an extrapolation of the results from one hospital to the rest of the NHS, which make it very difficult to derive an exact estimate. Nevertheless, this is the only estimate currently available. On the basis that infection control teams believe a reduction of 15 per cent is achievable, this suggests that potential avoidable costs are around £150 million a year (this excludes the cost of measures that might be needed to achieve this and assumes achievable reductions are across the full range of infections).

17   A large proportion of infection control teams said they would like to spend less time being reactive and spend more time on planned surveillance activities. Research shows that surveillance, involving data collection, analysis and feedback of results to clinicians is central to detecting infections, dealing with them, and ultimately reducing infection rates.

18   In general, surveillance needs to be done more effectively. While over 90 per cent of infection control teams had carried out some limited surveillance, there was a lack of comparable data on rates and trends. This limits the ability of NHS Trusts to have a good understanding of infection problems, both within the Trust and in comparison with other Trusts, and the effectiveness of any intervention measures employed. There were wide variations in the extent of dissemination of surveillance results.

19   The Nosocomial Infection National Surveillance Scheme, developed in 1996, is starting to show the benefits of surveillance. By December 1999, 139 hospitals had participated in one or more modules of the scheme. The scheme's first full year results show there is considerable scope for NHS Trusts to reduce infection rates through better practice. NHS Trusts surveyed reported a number of benefits of participating, but also problems that need to be overcome if the scheme is to be fully effective, in particular the need for an improvement in the feedback of results to NHS Trusts and, within NHS Trusts, to clinicians and senior managers.

20   Several studies have indicated that between 50 and 70 per cent of surgical wound infections occur post-discharge and the preliminary results from a comprehensive study in three NHS Trusts would appear to support these findings. However, only a quarter of infection control teams are carrying out any post-discharge surveillance.

21   While there is clearly scope to reduce hospital acquired infection, there will inevitably be an irreducible minimum. However, attempts to achieve this may be offset by NHS Trusts' bed management policies and developments whereby staff and patients move freely between wards. While there may be good reasons for this, it is important that the implications for hospital acquired infection are carefully considered as part of NHS Trusts' other policies.

Effectiveness of prevention, detection and control measures

22   There are wide variations in infection control teams' input into the main prevention, detection and control activities. The key activities include the provision of education and training; development and dissemination of infection control policies; monitoring and audit of hospital hygiene; and clinical audit.

23   It appears that there are important gaps in the extent to which education and training in infection control is provided to key health care staff. For example, currently some 10 per cent of infection control teams do not provide nurses and health care assistants with induction training about infection control and less than two thirds provide annual updates. Most teams do not provide any infection control training to senior doctors. The development of interactive computer assisted training packages could be a cost-effective way of helping to address the weaknesses in training and education.

24   Written infection control policies and procedures need to be more widely available and accessible. All NHS Trusts had policies in place for dealing with MRSA (methicillin resistant *Staphylococcus aureus* - an antibiotic resistant organism that is causing problems in most hospitals), patient isolation, handling of sharps such as disposable needles, and clinical waste management. But over a quarter of NHS Trusts did not have written policies for the use of catheters and other devices implicated in hospital acquired infections. Many infection control teams consider that producing and updating policies and guidelines, often as part of an infection control manual, is very time consuming. There is evidence of re-inventing the wheel and scope to streamline the production of infection control manuals.

25 Some eight per cent of NHS Trusts do not have a policy on handwashing. Handwashing is regarded by many as one of the most effective preventative measures against hospital acquired infection, and is one example of good practice that needs to be more widely implemented. There is ample evidence that compliance with handwashing protocols is poor. It is welcome that in March 1999, an NHS action plan was issued by the Department which included advice reinforcing the importance of handwashing.

26 Monitoring hospitals' routine procedures such as ward cleaning is important to ensure that proper hygiene practices are being followed and that they are working as intended. We found that most NHS Trusts had carried out such audits within the last three years. The results showed that NHS Trusts had made changes in response to audit reports, but in some there was scope for considerable improvement.

27 Infection control teams have a responsibility for standard setting and audit. Only 50 per cent of infection control teams included clinical audit in their annual infection control programme, though most acknowledged that it is an important part of the audit cycle to improve infection control. Eighty one per cent of infection control teams had not audited their own activities. In the last year, the main focus of audit attention was on arrangements for controlling MRSA, surgical wound audit, and antibiotic prescribing. A number of infection control teams identified interventions that had reduced particular infections and achieved cost savings, and which could be applied more widely.

28 Infection control has implications for the whole hospital and the advice of the infection control team is important in ensuring that the risk of infection is minimised. While around 50 per cent of infection control teams said they were usually consulted, a quarter were never consulted on the letting of cleaning, or catering or laundry contracts. While about half of infection control teams are usually consulted when an NHS Trust is contemplating alterations or additions to buildings, they are less likely to be consulted by staff purchasing equipment.

29 Well documented procedures for dealing with outbreaks of infection are essential, and all infection control teams had them. But about a quarter of infection control teams did not comply with the requirements for disseminating written reports to appropriate personnel within the Trust.

30 Screening patients for infections, which involves taking swabs from the patient and submitting them to microbiology testing, is one way of detecting some infections and controlling their spread. It is expensive to do, however, and there is little evidence on its cost effectiveness. The benefits of screening staff are even less certain, and also need to be further researched.

31 Evidence to the House of Lords Select Committee on Science and Technology inquiry on 'Resistance to Antibiotics and other Antimicrobial Agents' states that "Isolation of patients is an expensive, but effective form of infection control." There is, however, a lack of evidence based research on how best and when to use isolation facilities cost effectively. The number of isolation facilities within individual NHS Trusts have been greatly reduced over the last five years and over 40 per cent of infection control teams were dissatisfied with the facilities available in their Trust. Some 150 NHS Trusts have yet to assess the need for and provision of isolation facilities, regarded by the Department as part of risk assessments needed to meet Health and Safety legislation.

Recommendations for improving strategic management

32 We found that some NHS Trusts have put infection control high on their agenda and there was also evidence of good practice where infection control teams had made great efforts to overcome staffing and other resource constraints. The Department's positive response to the House of Lords Select Committee inquiry should go some way towards improving the strategic management of hospital acquired infection, as should the new infection control standards for acute NHS hospitals, recently issued as part of their new guidelines for implementing Controls Assurance in the NHS. However, we have identified areas where Acute NHS Trusts can improve the strategic management of infection control still further.

The Department should:

(i) consider the need for a revision of their 1995 guidance on infection control and ensure that the implementation of the controls assurance standard on infection control is monitored through the NHS performance management process and through the Commission for Health Improvement and the Audit Commission;

(ii) consider commissioning research on appropriate staffing levels for the infection control team, to help NHS Trusts determine an appropriate level of resources; and

Part 1: Background

Introduction

1.1   A hospital acquired infection is one that is neither present nor incubating at the time when a patient is admitted to hospital. We carried out a study of the management and control of hospital acquired infection because:

- at any given time, some 9 per cent of patients in hospital have a hospital acquired infection that can add to the patient's discomfort and length of stay and may adversely affect the treatment of the patient's original medical condition. It can result in prolonged or permanent disability and a small proportion of patients die;

- hospital-acquired infection may be costing the National Health Service as much as £1 billion a year;

- hospital acquired infection cannot be completely eradicated but, in 1995, the Hospital Infection Working Group of the Department of Health (Department) and Public Health Laboratory Service believed that about 30 per cent could be prevented;

- the House of Lords Select Committee on Science and Technology's report on "Resistance to Antibiotics and other Antimicrobial Agents" highlighted concerns about hospitals' infection control arrangements.

- hospital hygiene and infection control encompasses the whole NHS health care system;

- there is scope for improving infection control and our findings can promote greater awareness of the problem and better practice.

1.2   An infection occurs when a micro-organism (bacterium, a protozoan, a virus or a fungus) invades a susceptible host. The majority of hospital acquired infections are caused by bacteria. The most common are those affecting the urinary tract, surgical wounds, the lower respiratory tract, skin and the bloodstream[1]. Together they account for three quarters of all hospital acquired infections (see Figure 1). Less common causes include specific infectious diseases, like influenza and viral gastro-enteritis and in some very rare cases, infections such as Legionnaires disease and tuberculosis. Some infections are spread from person to person, some are derived from the patients own normal flora, while others may be the result of environmental contamination (for example legionella in water systems).[2]

Around 9 per cent of patients have a hospital acquired infection at any one time

The main sites of hospital acquired infections

Figure 1

Urinary tract infections are the most common type of hospital acquired infection and blood stream infections have the highest associated mortality

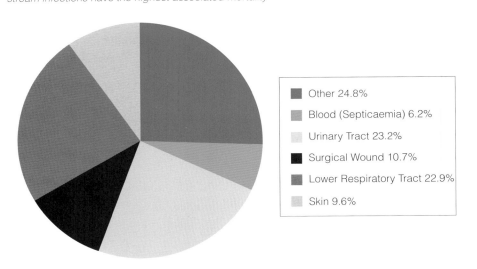

- Other 24.8%
- Blood (Septicaemia) 6.2%
- Urinary Tract 23.2%
- Surgical Wound 10.7%
- Lower Respiratory Tract 22.9%
- Skin 9.6%

Source: Second prevalence study Emmerson et al (1996)

Note: 37,111 patients from 15 centres were studied over a 15 month period from May 1993 to July 1994 in two month study periods and a mean hospital acquired infection prevalence rate of 9% (range 2-29%) was calculated.[1]

1.3 There is no requirement for NHS Trusts to publish data on hospital acquired infection and such data that have been published are not comparable. While most NHS Trusts undertake some form of surveillance to detect hospital acquired infection, there are wide variations in the methods used, types of infection monitored, ways infection rates are measured and criteria used for defining infections. However, two national prevalence surveys published in the United Kingdom in 1981[3] and 1996[1] found that, at any one time, 9 per cent of patients were suffering from an infection acquired after their admission to hospital.

1.4 Though there were methodological and other differences between the surveys, 9 per cent is widely quoted as the prevalence of hospital acquired infection in the United Kingdom. In both studies, the overall prevalence figures mask considerable variations in different patient groups with prevalence greatest in intensive care patients and higher in surgical patients than medical patients. Prevalence studies in other countries over the last 20 years tend to show similar levels of hospital acquired infection[4], though reliable international comparisons are difficult to make.

1.5 A 1992 study (Glenister et al)[5] examined the incidence of hospital acquired infection occurring in patients admitted to medical, surgical, urology, gynaecology and orthopaedic units at one district general hospital during a thirteen month period. The overall incidence was 9.2 per cent. As with prevalence studies the overall rate concealed the wide variations in infection rates between the different hospital specialities. These ranged from 7.2 per cent in the medical speciality to 13.4 per cent of patients in the orthopaedic speciality. Similar incidence rates were found in a study, conducted between August 1994 and September 1995, into the control of hospital acquired infection in nineteen hospitals in England and Wales[6]. The results of this study suggested that there may be at least 100,000 cases of hospital acquired infection each year.

1.6 None of the studies mentioned above took into account hospital acquired infections that develop after a patient leaves hospital. With moves towards shorter hospital stays, the number of infections that manifest themselves post-discharge is likely to be growing, but few NHS Trusts are aware of their post discharge infection rates. Several studies have indicated that between 50 and 70 per cent of surgical wound infections occur post-discharge[7]. This suggests that the true extent of hospital acquired infection is higher than the prevalence or incidence studies suggest.

Some patients die each year as a result of hospital acquired infections

1.7 In the mid1980's in the United States of America, it was estimated that hospital acquired infection was amongst the top ten causes of death if cases where hospital acquired infection was a substantial contributor were added to cases where it was the primary cause (Haley, et al)[8]. The Department's 1995 guidance on the control of infection in hospitals, issued under (HSG(95)10)[9] as Departmental policy on infection control, noted that "equivalent data are not available in the UK, and, whilst accepting the difficulties of extrapolating from one system of health care to another, ... a crude comparison indicates that if US rates were applicable in the United Kingdom, 5,000 deaths (1 per cent of all deaths) might be primarily attributable to hospital acquired infection and in a further 15,000 cases (3 per cent of all deaths) hospital acquired infection might be a substantial contributor." The guidance acknowledges that "many deaths from hospital acquired infection occur in patients already dying from other causes and/or in patients whose infection were not preventable. Nevertheless, the numbers are very large and a proportion of these deaths is avoidable".

Hospital acquired infection is becoming harder to treat

1.8   Antibiotics have been used successfully for more than 50 years to control, and in many instances overcome bacterial infections. While antibiotics have proved useful in the treatment of infection, their use has led to the emergence of highly resistant strains of bacteria (Figure 2). These drug resistant infections are commonest in hospitals where high levels of antibiotic usage allow organisms to evolve, and the close concentration of people with increased susceptibility to infection allows the organisms to spread.

1.9   The 1998 House of Lords Select Committee report on Resistance to Antibiotics and other Antimicrobial Agents (House of Lords Report)[10] identified growing concerns about the rise of MRSA (methicillin resistant *Staphylococcus aureus*) and other hospital infections. They noted that this is a worldwide problem and that levels of MRSA in this country are low by international standards. However, they are rising. They concluded that MRSA poses one of the biggest challenges to infection control, and that in many hospitals it is now endemic.

Figure 2	Examples of types of emergent resistant strains of bacteria

Staphylococcus aureus is one of the most common of all bacteria. About one-third of the population carry it on the skin, or in the nose and throat. However, if the bacteria enter the body, for instance through a surgical wound, they can cause

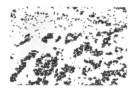

serious infections such as septicaemia or pneumonia. Methicillin resistant *Staphylococcus aureus* (MRSA) is an antibiotic resistant variety of the bacterium. There are epidemic strains of MRSA which spread very readily from person to person. It is a common cause of outbreaks, necessitating temporary closure of wards and disrupting hospital services. A total of 189 hospitals in England and Wales are known to have had incidents of MRSA in 1995. By 1998 it was a problem in most hospitals, indeed in 1998 there were 1597 incidents of MRSA (where an incident is defined as 3 or more patients with the same strain in the same hospital in one calendar month).

Enterococci bacteria are part of the normal flora of the human gut. If the organisms gain access to normally sterile parts of the body in vulnerable patients such as kidney dialysis and bone-marrow transplant patients they

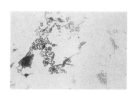

can cause a range of different types of infection. Serious infections can be extremely difficult to treat because the bacteria are often innately resistant to all "standard" antibiotics. The emergence of Glycopeptide resistant *enterococci* (GRE) is a cause of particular concern because of the fear that the genetic material which carries the resistance may transfer into MRSA (making MRSA virtually untreatable). GRE infections are as yet relatively uncommon. However, Glycopeptide intermediate MRSA strains have been isolated in Japan, the US and Scotland.

Hospital acquired infection may be costing the NHS as much as £1 billion each year

1.10 Treating a hospital acquired infection imposes an additional burden on the hospital and may also result in additional costs to general practitioners, district nursing services, and a range of other health care and community services. Studies that have estimated the economic burden of hospital acquired infection generally limit the range of costs examined to those that fall on the hospital sector.[11] The main factors contributing to the direct costs of treating hospital acquired infections are increased length of stay and additional antibiotic therapy and, where necessary, the need for repeat surgery. Identifying these costs requires surveillance of infection rates, measurement of extended length of stay and detailed costing of therapies. However, most of the available information relates to specific infections or prevention measures rather than to overall costs, and the estimates derived vary considerably.

1.11 Some NHS Trusts have attempted to cost individual outbreaks of hospital acquired infection. These costs can be large. For example, a two year outbreak of MRSA in Kettering was estimated to have cost the hospital £400,000[9], see Case Study 1. These costs do not include the cost of additional length of stay, additional prescribing costs or absence from work of staff colonised with MRSA.

Case Study 1

Cost of MRSA outbreak in Kettering in 1991-92

Isolation wards	£303,600
Microbiology	£ 43,000
Drugs	£ 17,100
Cleaning	£ 25,600
Replacement of mattresses and pillows	£ 6,800
Community nurse	£ 7,500
Total (i)	£403,600

Source: Data from Cox et al - Journal of Hospital Infection (1995) 29, 87-106 - as presented in the Department's Guidance on the control of infections in hospital[9]

1.12 In 1994, the Department commissioned the London School of Hygiene and Tropical Medicine and Public Health Laboratory Service to develop a model to cost the socio-economic impact of hospital acquired infection. The study patients were recruited from one district general hospital and the results were extrapolated by the researchers to calculate national estimates of the economic burden of hospital acquired infection. The report, which was published in January 2000[12] shows that the impact of hospital acquired infection on NHS hospitals is considerable (Figure 3).

1.13 The results show that the additional cost of hospital acquired infection incurred by adult non-day case patients who acquired an infection in the study hospital was £3.6 million. The total gross costs to NHS hospitals was estimated at £930 million or 9.1% of the inpatient programme budget. In addition, a further £55.7 million was estimated to have been incurred post discharge by GPs, outpatient consultants and district nursing services. Extrapolating results from the one hospital in this study to the rest of the NHS is very difficult. The Department does not believe it is possible to derive an accurate estimate of the overall cost to the NHS on the basis of the experience of one hospital. However, this is the only estimate of costs currently available and more evidence based research needs to be done in this area.

**Key findings from the
study of the
socio-economic burden of
hospital acquired
infection**

Figure 3

■ Over the course of a 13 month period, 7.8% of patients acquired an infection during their stay in the study hospital which presented during the in-patient period.

■ A further 19.1% of patients who did not present with an infection during the in-patient phase, reported symptoms of, and in some cases received treatment for, an infection manifesting post discharge which may be associated with their hospital admission.

■ Patients with one or more infections incurred costs that were on average 2.8 times greater than uninfected patients, an average additional cost of £2,917 per case (ranging from £1,122 for urinary tract infections to £6,209 for bloodstream infections).

■ Patients who acquired an infection remained in hospital on average 2.5 times longer than uninfected patients, an average equivalent to 11 extra days.

■ Patients with a hospital acquired infection were 7.1 times more likely to die in the hospital than uninfected patients (after controlling for patient characteristics such as age, sex, diagnosis, admission speciality and type and pre-exiting illness). The death rate also varied with patient characteristics (for example 38% of elderly care patients who acquired a hospital infection died compared with 8% of elderly patients without a hospital acquired infection who died).

Source: *Study by the London
School of Hygiene and Tropical
Medicine and Public Health
Laboratory Service*[12]

■ Extrapolating the results of this study to NHS Trusts throughout England, the overall cost to the NHS of hospital acquired infection was £986.36 million comprising £930.62 million hospital costs plus a further £55.74 million costs due to infections which occurred post discharge.

Hospital acquired infection cannot be eradicated but a proportion may be avoidable

1.14 Not all hospital acquired infection is preventable nor is it likely to become so in the foreseeable future. The very old and the very young, who have less efficient or immature immune systems, are particularly susceptible to hospital infections, as are patients undergoing therapies that suppress the immune system, such as transplant patients, chemotherapy patients, and patients with diseases affecting the immune system. The length of stay in hospital is a risk factor and so are severity of illness, use of invasive procedures and presence of medical devices. The London School of Hygiene and Tropical Medicine and Public Health Laboratory Service report[12] noted that although a shorter hospital stay will reduce the risk of acquiring an infection, for surgical patients the risk is likely to be highest on the day of surgery and the days immediately following.

1.15 The Department's 1995 guidance[9] acknowledged that the proportion of infections that were preventable varied according to the characteristics of the group of patients involved. Also that some types of infections were more serious for the patient than others and that efforts to prevent them were more likely to repay the investment required. However, the Hospital Infection Working Group, responsible for preparing the guidance, believed that

> "it is possible that currently about 30 per cent of hospital acquired infection could be prevented by better application of existing knowledge and implementation of realistic infection control policies".

The guidance recognised that infection control action would be constrained by the resources available but that efforts to prevent or control outbreaks were likely to save significant sums in the longer term.

1.16 The Department's guidance illustrated the point using the results from the American SENIC study (Haley et al)[8] which showed that hospitals with infection control programmes that included surveillance and feedback of results to clinicians reduced infections by 32%. The guidance noted that in the 1970's when the American study was carried out, routine infection control activities were not well established in many hospitals there and that in the United Kingdom in the 1990s it may not be possible to achieve such dramatic results. Nevertheless, this demonstrates that there is scope for improving quality of patient care and health outcomes.

The NHS management framework for the control of hospital acquired infection

1.17 The management of hospital acquired infection is complex. Figure 4 details the responsibilities within the NHS. The Department has overall policy responsibility and the chief executive of every hospital NHS Trust is responsible for ensuring that effective infection control arrangements are in place and subject to regular review. The key management forum for infection control within NHS Trusts is the Hospital Infection Control Committee, and all acute hospitals should have an infection control team, which has primary responsibility for all aspects of surveillance, prevention and control of infection at NHS Trust level.[9]

Figure 4   **Responsibilities in the NHS in relation to hospital acquired infection**

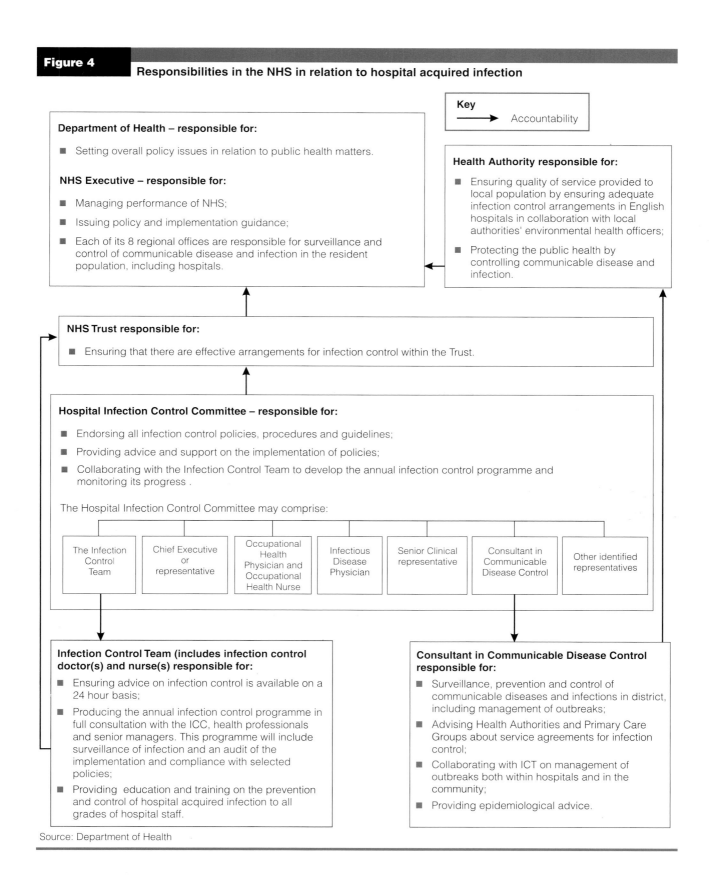

Key
→ Accountability

Department of Health – responsible for:

■ Setting overall policy issues in relation to public health matters.

NHS Executive – responsible for:

■ Managing performance of NHS;

■ Issuing policy and implementation guidance;

■ Each of its 8 regional offices are responsible for surveillance and control of communicable disease and infection in the resident population, including hospitals.

Health Authority responsible for:

■ Ensuring quality of service provided to local population by ensuring adequate infection control arrangements in English hospitals in collaboration with local authorities' environmental health officers;

■ Protecting the public health by controlling communicable disease and infection.

NHS Trust responsible for:

■ Ensuring that there are effective arrangements for infection control within the Trust.

Hospital Infection Control Committee – responsible for:

■ Endorsing all infection control policies, procedures and guidelines;

■ Providing advice and support on the implementation of policies;

■ Collaborating with the Infection Control Team to develop the annual infection control programme and monitoring its progress .

The Hospital Infection Control Committee may comprise:

| The Infection Control Team | Chief Executive or representative | Occupational Health Physician and Occupational Health Nurse | Infectious Disease Physician | Senior Clinical representative | Consultant in Communicable Disease Control | Other identified representatives |

Infection Control Team (includes infection control doctor(s) and nurse(s) responsible for:

■ Ensuring advice on infection control is available on a 24 hour basis;

■ Producing the annual infection control programme in full consultation with the ICC, health professionals and senior managers. This programme will include surveillance of infection and an audit of the implementation and compliance with selected policies;

■ Providing education and training on the prevention and control of hospital acquired infection to all grades of hospital staff.

Consultant in Communicable Disease Control responsible for:

■ Surveillance, prevention and control of communicable diseases and infections in district, including management of outbreaks;

■ Advising Health Authorities and Primary Care Groups about service agreements for infection control;

■ Collaborating with ICT on management of outbreaks both within hospitals and in the community;

■ Providing epidemiological advice.

Source: Department of Health

1.18 In addition, since 1988, each health authority has been required to appoint at least one Consultant in Communicable Disease Control to maintain a balanced perspective on the wider issues of infection control (Acheson Report on Public Health, England[13]). Consultants in Communicable Disease Control are responsible for the surveillance, prevention and control of communicable diseases and infection within a district health authority. In addition they are:

- members of a NHS Trust's Hospital Infection Control Committee;

- required to provide hospitals with epidemiological advice and ensure the wider community perspectives of infection control are understood;

- expected to collaborate with the infection control team in managing infection outbreaks; and

- often appointed as "Proper Officer" for the control of infectious diseases within a local authority under the Public Health (Control of Diseases) Act 1984 for which they are accountable to local authorities.

The components of good infection control

1.19 In addition to the need for an effective management framework, the Department's 1995 Guidance[9] and the 1993 Standards in Infection Control in Hospitals[14] detail the key components of an effective infection control regime which infection control teams are advised to follow (Figure 5). In 1997 and 1999 the Department reminded health authorities and NHS Trusts of the need to ensure that appropriate arrangements for communicable disease surveillance and control were in place.[15, 17]

The main components of an effective infection control programme

Figure 5

The main components include:

- Surveillance of infection - to produce accurate timely information on infection rates and trends, detect outbreaks, inform evaluations of and changes in clinical practice, and assist the targeting of preventative efforts.

- Provision of education and training - to inform and convince staff of the value of recommended infection control measures.

- Production, review and dissemination of written policies, procedures and guidelines on the NHS Trust's infection control arrangements.

- Monitoring of hospital hygiene - in relation to cleaning, housekeeping, disinfection or sterilisation of instruments and equipment, safe collection and disposal of clinical waste; kitchen hygiene etc.

- Setting and auditing standards of own work, and contributing to the standard setting and audit processes in other clinical and support services to ensure compliance with infection control policies and procedures.

- Contributing to decisions on: the purchase of equipment; plans for alterations and additions to the building; and the letting of catering, domestic and laundry services contracts.

- Specific documented arrangements for dealing with infections, including outbreak control, targeted screening and isolation of patients.

Source: Department of Health Guidance on Control of Infections in Hospital (HSG (95)10)[9]

A national surveillance scheme has been developed to improve patient care by providing local and national data on infection rates

1.20 Surveillance is the key component of the infection control programme and the effectiveness of the other prevention, detection and control measures is improved if they are underpinned by an effective surveillance strategy. Since 1996, the Department and the Public Health Laboratory Service have been working together to develop a national surveillance scheme (the Nosocomial Infection National Surveillance Scheme). The aim of the scheme is to improve patient care by providing information to assist NHS Trusts to reduce rates and risk of hospital acquired infection and to provide national statistics on specific types of infection for comparison with local results.

1.21 Although there are some limitations to the Nosocomial Infection National Surveillance Scheme as it is currently operated, namely the fact that it comprises self-selected hospitals, the first years data provides the most comprehensive set of comparable data available to the NHS.[16] In addition to giving some indication of national rates for specific specialities and types of operation, the results allow individual hospitals participating in the scheme to compare their own performance with the national rates. By December 1999, the number of hospitals which had participated in one or more 3 month modules, had grown to 139. Over time, the data collected will also permit analysis of trends in hospital acquired infection and should enable NHS Trusts to target their infection control activities to maximum effect.

Other steps are being taken to address hospital acquired infection

1.22 Since 1988, the Department has taken a number of initiatives to address hospital acquired infection (Figure 6). As a result the profile given to infection control by the Government and the Department, particularly in the last two years has increased significantly. For example, the Department emphasised the importance of infection control in the National Priorities Guidance for 1999-2002.[17] Also the Government's response [Cm 4172 December 1998] to the House of Lord's Report (HL Paper 81-1)[18], noted that infection control is at the heart of the quality of clinical care provided by hospitals, also that:

■ performance indicators and/or targets on hospital infection control, including MRSA, need to be introduced, and that the development of robust indicators to provide this information is underway; and

■ the Department is working with the Public Health Laboratory Service to identify ways to improve its surveillance as part of a new overall surveillance strategy for antimicrobial resistance.

Key Department of Health initiatives to address hospital acquired infection

Figure 6

■ In 1988, a Joint Working Group set up by the then Department of Health and Social Security and the Public Health Laboratory Service produced the first national guidance on infection control in hospitals, including the need to establish Infection Control Committees and infection control teams.

■ In 1993, an Infection Control Standards Working Group comprising the Association of Medical Microbiologists, Hospital Infection Society, Infection Control Nurses Association and Public Health Laboratory Service, issued "Standards in Infection Control in Hospitals". While not issued by the Department of Health, the standards were acknowledged by them as providing a suitable framework for infection control teams to follow.

■ In March 1995, the Hospital Infection Working Group of the Department and Public Health Laboratory service issued revised Hospital Infection Control Guidance. The guidance, known as the Cooke Report, was issued under cover of HSG(95) 10 with the statement that this was "now Department of Health policy on infection control". This guidance strengthened the 1988 guidance and included new advice on improving surveillance of hospital acquired infection.

continued…

Key Department of Health initiatives to address hospital acquired infection *continued*

Figure 6

- In March 1996, the Department of Health and Public Health Laboratory Service established the Nosocomial Infection National Surveillance Scheme to improve patient care by helping hospitals to reduce rates and risk of hospital acquired infection. This was the first attempt to produce national data on hospital acquired infection for comparison with local results. The first Annual Reports on surgical site infections was published in December 1999. A report on the first two years of bacteraemia results is expected to be published in 2000.

- In 1997, the Department commissioned regional epidemiologists to examine communicable disease control services provided by local health authorities throughout England. The survey identified a number of shortcomings and that communicable disease control was hard pressed in some areas. The results of this study have been considered by Regional Offices and action is being taken to address identified shortcomings.

- In 1997 and 1998, the Government's NHS Priorities and Planning Guidance made it clear that health authorities must satisfy themselves that appropriate arrangements are in place for communicable disease control. In particular, the "National Priorities Guidance for 1999/00 – 2001-02" (HSC(98)159: LAC(98)22), issued in September 1998, required health authorities to ensure "continuing and effective protection of the public health with particular regard to the prevention and control of hospital infection, communicable diseases, antibiotic resistance and the effects of environmental and chemical hazards".

- In February 1998, the Department commissioned the production of evidence-based guidelines on the general principles for preventing hospital acquired infections. The guidelines which contain many elements of clinical practice for preventing the spread of hospital acquired infection, including multi-drug resistant organisms, are expected to be completed in Summer 2000. The project has been extended and guidelines have been commissioned for the prevention and control of infection in primary and community care settings.

- In June 1998, the Department commissioned regional epidemiologists to examine infection control arrangements in NHS Trusts. The results of this study have been considered by Regional Directors of Public Health and an action plan is being taken forward to address areas where shortcomings were identified.

- In September 1998, following a request from the then Chief Medical Officer, the Standing Medical Advisory Committee (SMAC) produced its report "The Path of Least Resistance". The report examined antimicrobial resistance in relation to medical prescribing. The report stressed that effective infection control was fundamental to preventing the spread of resistant organisms.

- In December 1998, in response to the House of Lords report, the Government re-affirmed that infection control and hygiene should be a core management responsibility.

- In 1998, health protection arrangements were considered as part of the Chief Medical Officer's project to strengthen the public health function. One of the main recommendations was the development of a communicable disease strategy and work on this is in progress.

- In March 1999, the Department issued HSC 1999/049 detailing action for the NHS following the Government's response to the House of Lords report and the SMAC report, the "Path of Least Resistance". Regional Offices are in the process of implementing action plans.

continued...

Key Department of Health initiatives to address hospital acquired infection

Figure 6

- In May 1999, as part of Governance in the new NHS, the Department issued HSC 1999/123 setting out action for NHS Trusts and health authorities for 1999-2000 in respect of moving beyond financial controls assurance statements to the production of statements covering wider organisational controls, including risk management.

- In November 1999, the Department issued further guidance, supplementing HSC 1999/123. New risk management and organisational standards, including controls assurance standards for infection control, were launched and sent out to the NHS.

- In December 1999, the Government published 'Modernising Health and Social Services: National Priorities Guidance 2000-01 and 2002-03'. This stressed the importance of working in partnership and required the NHS to "strengthen services to prevent and control communicable diseases, especially hospital acquired infection, taking action to reduce antimicrobial resistance..." (HSC(99)242:LAC(99)38.

Source: Department of Health

1.23 There is now a substantial agenda of work in place designed to assure and improve the quality of health care provided by the NHS. Clinical governance is central to this[19]. It provides all NHS organisations and health care professionals with a framework which, over the next five years, will develop into a coherent local programme for clinical quality improvement. The main components of clinical governance are: clear lines of accountability and responsibility; a comprehensive programme of quality improvement activities, such as clinical audit; clear policies aimed at managing risk; and procedures for all professional groups to identify and remedy poor performance. Clinical governance interfaces with a number of other key strategic developments, such as the Commission for Health Improvement. As part of its functions, the Commission for Health Improvement will review and monitor the implementation of clinical governance.

1.24 The new standards for the control of infection in acute NHS Trusts issued by the Department in November 1999, are part of the framework for managing risk and levelling up standards in the NHS. NHS Trusts are required to assess their performance against national standards of good practice, including establishing effective management structures and responsibilities, setting indicators to demonstrate improvements in infection control and providing training to all health care staff in infection control. NHS Trusts are required to assess themselves against the standards by March 2000 and set out plans to implement the measures to meet the requirements by July 2000. Progress will be monitored locally by auditors and nationally by the Commission for Health Improvement and the Audit Commission.

Other services and statutory bodies have a role in ensuring that NHS Trusts have an effective infection control regime

1.25 A number of other services routinely deal with issues around the practice of infection control within the NHS Trust. For example, the Trust occupational health services have a responsibility to advise managers and employees about the effect of work on health and health on work and to devise risk management programmes to ensure that hazards which staff face during their work are minimised. Close co-operation and liaison between the infection control team and occupational health staff is essential in formulating and implementing measures to avoid staff contracting or spreading infections in the course of their employment. Similarly, catering service managers are required to ensure that the hospital meets food safety legislation and other service managers such as estates managers, hotel services managers and operating theatre managers, have a role to play in liasing with the infection control team to ensure that the risk of transmission is minimised.

1.26 Other statutory agencies have a regulatory function in relation to the control of infection. For example the Health and Safety Executive is the enforcing agency for the Health and Safety at Work Act 1974 and the Control of Substances Hazardous to Health Regulations 1994. NHS Trusts are required to report to the Health and Safety Executive certain diseases and dangerous occurrences such as outbreaks of Legionnaires Disease.

Scope of the study

1.27 Against this background, we examined whether the overall management and control of hospital acquired infection in Acute NHS Trusts, is carried out in accordance with existing guidelines and standards. We have also considered whether infection control arrangements in these hospitals are effective and how they could be improved, and identified the factors constraining the application of existing knowledge and realistic infection control measures.

1.28 Our report considers:

■ strategic management of hospital acquired infection (Part 2);

■ surveillance and its effectiveness in reducing hospital acquired infection (Part 3); and

■ the effectiveness of infection control practices and procedures (Part 4).

Methodology

1.29 The main element of our methodology was a census of Acute NHS Trusts in England. The census was based on a self completion audit programme comprised of two questionnaires, completed by or on behalf of chief executives and the NHS Trust's infection control team respectively. We designed the audit programme to:

- test the extent of compliance with the Department's guidelines and standards, in particular the Department's 1995 guidance on the control of infection in hospitals[9];

- identify the impact of infection control arrangements within individual NHS Trusts; and

- identify examples of good practice.

1.30 The audit programme was piloted at seven NHS Trusts before despatch to all 219 Acute NHS Trusts in England. All NHS Trusts eventually returned their completed audit programme. A more detailed description of the areas covered by the audit programme and types of analyses used to evaluate the results is at Appendix 1.

1.31 In addition we:

- reviewed published literature on extent and cost of hospital acquired infection and good practice;

- obtained detailed information and data from the Nosocomial Infection National Surveillance Scheme team, Public Health Laboratory Service and the London School of Hygiene and Tropical Medicine;

- reviewed literature on hospital infection control arrangements in other countries, and visited the Center for Disease Control and Prevention in Atlanta, USA, principally to review the operation of the American Nosocomial Infection National Surveillance System;

- attended a number of workshops and conferences, and consulted numerous interested parties including Royal Colleges; and

■ convened a panel of experts to assist us in study design and interpretation of results (Appendix 1, paragraph 14).

Feedback to NHS Trusts and liaison with the Department of Health

1.32 At the time of our census (July 1998) the Regional Directors of Public Health had already asked the regional epidemiologists, who provide advice and support to the NHS Executive on communicable disease matters, to carry out a survey of NHS acute Trusts' arrangements for hospital acquired infection. By mutual agreement and to avoid unnecessary duplication of effort we agreed to make our audit data available to the regional epidemiologists. NHS Trusts were informed of this in a joint letter from the Department of Health and the National Audit Office, prior to sending out the audit programmes.

1.33 Regional epidemiologists have analysed the data from the census on a regional and individual NHS Trust basis and have submitted their findings to Regional Directors of Public Health. They will consider these reports and take any action deemed necessary. Action plans are being developed by individual NHS Trusts to improve the Trust's approach to the management and control of hospital acquired infection. In addition to this National Audit Office report, we have provided a short report to each NHS Trust that participated in the survey, detailing how their performance on several key areas compares with the national picture.

Part 2: Strategic management of hospital acquired infection

2.1 The Department's guidance requires the chief executive of every NHS Trust to ensure that effective infection control arrangements are in place. Managerial interest at a strategic level and commitment and support of senior management and heads of clinical directorates is essential. This part of the report examines the strategic management of infection control. It considers the overall priority given to hospital infection control in NHS Trusts and evaluates the staffing and other resources available to implement infection control activities.

The relationship between Health Authorities and NHS Trusts

2.2 Health Authorities are required to protect the public health by controlling communicable disease and infection. This responsibility includes ensuring adequate infection control arrangements within hospitals. The Department of Health's 1995[9] guidance stated that communicable disease control and infection should be taken into consideration in every contract which health authorities placed with acute hospitals. Under the Labour administration, long term service level agreements replaced contracts as the main basis for the relationship between health authorities and NHS Trusts. The NHS National Priorities and Planning Guidelines for 1999/00-2001/02[17] and Health Service Circular 1999/049[20] set out an action for the NHS following the Government's response[18] to the House of Lords Select Committee Report on Antibiotic Resistance.[10] This reminded Health Authorities, NHS Trusts and Primary Care Groups of their obligations to ensure:

■ the continuing and effective protection of the public's health, with particular regard to the prevention and control of hospital infection, communicable disease, and antibiotic resistance; and

■ that progress in meeting this commitment should be monitored locally through the normal performance management process.

Infection control is not covered as well as it should be in many NHS Trust's agreements with health authorities

2.3 The Department's 1995 guidance suggested that initially health authorities should concentrate on ensuring that an effective programme of surveillance and feedback was in place, supported by other activities to identify and address areas of concern. In particular the priority should be on the development of year on year comparisons of surveillance data within the hospital.

2.4 We found that three-quarters of NHS Trusts had contracts with their health authorities that covered the provision of infection control services. Of these, a number met the main requirements of the guidelines. For example, 104 contracts (66%) specified the need to undertake surveillance, and 43 (27%) stated the need to calculate infection rates and supply this information to the health authority. Case Study 2 is an example of a contract that meets the main requirements of the guidance.

Case study 2

Coverage of infection control in the Quality Specification in the 1994/95 contract between Manchester Health Authority and North Manchester NHS Healthcare Trust

The contract covered two main aspects with regard to infection control. The NHS Trust was required to demonstrate to the purchaser that management procedures were in place to ensure the effective control of infection within the hospital and that it was developing effective, on-going methods of improving control of infection in the hospital.

The contract required the North Manchester Healthcare NHS Trust to provide the following information to Manchester Health Authority:

- A description of the management structure for the control of infection and of the system in place to ensure all staff are aware of the role and responsibilities of the Infection Control Team.
- A list of all policies that are in place that support infection control.
- A description of the routine infection surveillance undertaken with the results of that surveillance reported six monthly.
- Details of audit projects in infection control planned for the contractual year.
- A description of the education and training programme including who is trained and the number of staff trained.
- An end of year report of audits of infection control including all changes in practice implemented as a result of the audit.

The Consultant in Communicable Disease Control for the Health Authority was consulted in drawing up the contract. He is a member of the Hospital Infection Control Committee and advises the Health Authority on compliance with the contract. Both the NHS Trust and the Health Authority believe the contract arrangements have helped to improve the overall profile and approach to infection control.

2.5 For contracts/service agreements to be effective, the process of determining the infection control specifications within them should ideally involve personnel with detailed knowledge of infectious disease, that is the Consultant in Communicable Disease Control, the Infection Control Doctor and Infection Control Nurse. A 1997 survey commissioned by Regional Directors of Public Health[22] noted that the regional epidemiologists' assessment of markers of good practice included the observation that, within health authorities, "only 60 per cent of Consultants in Communicable Disease Control had adequate input into the contracting process; and 19 per cent had unsatisfactory arrangements."

2.6 The Economic and Social Research Council, Risk and Human Behaviour Programme, funded a study undertaken by the Health Services Research Unit at the London School of Hygiene and Tropical Medicine to determine how risks associated with infections and the control of infectious diseases are managed and distributed in the NHS[23]. This included how risks of infectious diseases were handled in formal agreements between health authorities and NHS Trusts. The findings from their survey of Consultants in Communicable Disease Control, infection control doctors and infection control nurses, which was conducted in December 1998–March 1999, confirmed the finding from our survey that requirements for infection control were not always included in the service agreements. Also, that even where they were included, fewer than one in five infection control doctors and just under a half of the Consultants in Communicable Disease Control were involved in developing the infection control specification.

2.7 We visited eight Consultants in Communicable Disease Control who told us that, to their knowledge, there was generally limited monitoring within the health authority of NHS Trust's compliance with the contract's infection control requirements.

2.8 The lack of information and compliance with the guidance on service agreements means that many health authorities do not have all the data on hospital acquired infections they need to assess NHS Trusts' performance in improving infection control. It also means that the opportunity to secure an appropriate standard of service may be missed. We conclude, as did the House of Lords Select Committee in March 1998 (HL Paper 81-I, 7th Report, Session 1997-98),[10] that there is considerable scope for health authorities to improve their service agreements and relationships with NHS Trusts to ensure that hospital infection control arrangements are robust and comply with good practice guidelines and standards. We note that the NHS Executive in its action plan (HSC 1999/049)[20], in response to the House of Lords Select Committee Report on Antibiotic Resistance[10] emphasised the importance of health authorities and NHS Trusts ensuring that infection control and basic hygiene are put at the heart of good management and clinical practice. We consider that this should involve a review of their service agreements, with input from the Consultant in Communicable Disease Control and Infection Control Team where this is currently lacking.

In many NHS Trusts infection control may not have the profile it merits

2.9 The Department's 1995 guidance[9] places responsibility for ensuring the provision of effective infection control arrangements on the hospital chief executive. This responsibility was reinforced in the Governments response to the House of Lords report.[18] The main requirements specified in the guidance are that the chief executive should:

■ formally approve the infection control programme;

■ receive regular progress reports of important incidents, lessons learned and surveillance and audit results, following discussion at the Hospital Infection Control Committee meeting; and

■ receive an annual report on the infection control programme, indicating achievements and drawing attention to any matters of concern;

2.10 To obtain an overview of chief executives' direct involvement in infection control in NHS Trusts we analysed the responses to seven questions in our survey. These questions, which were designed to test the chief executives' compliance with the above requirements in the Department's guidance, were scored on a simple Yes/No basis. Figure 7 shows that sixteen NHS Trusts scored zero while 87 (41 per cent) scored yes on four or more questions and only one scored yes on all seven questions. This analysis suggests that chief executives of most NHS Trusts are not as directly involved as the guidance suggests they should be.

Analysis of seven survey questions which give an overview of chief executives direct involvement in Infection Control in NHS Trusts

Figure 7

Overall, sixteen Trusts did not score on any of the questions indicating no direct chief executive involvement and only one Trust scored on all seven questions.

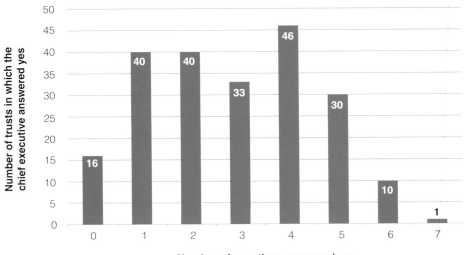

The 7 questions asked:

■ Is infection control discussed at Board meetings at least once a year?;

■ Does the Chief Executive receive minutes of HICC meetings?;

■ Does the Chief Executive receive the HICC annual report?;

■ Does the Chief Executive receive regular activity reports produced by the infection control team on the amount spent on hospital acquired infection at least annually?;

■ Does the Chief Executive receive regular activity reports produced by the infection control team on the rates of hospital acquired infection at least annually?;

■ Does the Chief Executive receive regular activity reports produced by the infection control team on the number of cases of hospital acquired infection at least annually?;

Source: NAO census ■ Does the Chief Executive formally approve the infection control programme?

2.11 Sixty seven per cent of chief executives receive the minutes of the Hospital Infection Control Committee and 45 per cent receive the Hospital Infection Control Committee annual report. However, only 43 per cent of chief executives receive any annual information on the rates, and 48 per cent on the number, of cases of hospital acquired infection. Fifty eight per cent of chief executives never receive an annual or more regular report on the amount spent on hospital acquired infection. This suggests that, in a number of NHS Trusts, chief executives may have a low level of awareness of infection control issues and that they may be unaware of the extent and cost of hospital acquired infection and how it is being addressed in their NHS Trust.

2.12 Infection control teams told us that the overall profile of infection control can be increased if it is a regular item on the Trust Board agenda. While 122 NHS Trusts (57 per cent) discussed infection control at the Trust Board at least once a year, 26 NHS Trusts (12 per cent) never discussed infection control at the Trust Board (15 NHS Trusts did not answer the question). In response to our survey findings the Department pointed out that while chief executives have overall responsibility for infection control this does not mean that they would necessarily expect to be involved directly in all aspects of its management. Also that chief executives routinely delegate matters which are formally their responsibility to other members of their senior management team. The answers to the questions addressed to the chief executive do not provide us with sufficient evidence to enable us to draw conclusions about the level of senior management involvement. Nevertheless, from visits to trusts and discussions with infection control teams we consider that, in many trusts, infection control may not have the profile it merits. The Department told us that the controls assurance standards, issued in November 1999, were one of the measures intended to address this issue.

There is a risk that some Hospital Infection Control Committees may not be fulfilling the role envisaged for them

2.13 The main forum for strategic and financial decisions for infection control is the Hospital Infection Control Committee (Committee). Departmental guidance[9] views the Committee as the main means of ensuring the collaboration and support of other hospital staff. In addition to the infection control team and representatives from various clinical and medical specialities, the chief executive or a nominated representative is expected to be a member of this Trust's Committee. All NHS Trusts in our survey, with the exception of a specialist homeopathic hospital, had a Committee.

2.14 Trust membership of the Committee varies as does the attendance of its members (Figure 8). For example, only 11 per cent of chief executives (22 NHS Trusts) are personally members of their Committee, and of these only 2 regularly attend meetings and 4 never attend. Chief Executives in about two thirds of NHS Trusts (138) have nominated a deputy to sit on the Committee and 90% of these generally attend the majority of meetings. However, in 64 NHS Trusts (30 per cent) neither the chief executive nor a nominated deputy sits on the Committee.

2.15 For infection control to be fully effective, a NHS Trust's occupational health service and the health authority's communicable disease function should be closely associated with the Trust's infection control service. The Committee is the forum to bring these functions together. Yet in 41 per cent of Trusts the Occupational Health Physician was not a member and in 19 per cent of Trusts the Consultant in Communicable Disease Control was not a member.

| **Figure 8** | Membership of NHS Trust's Hospital Infection Control Committees and frequency of attendance |

This shows that the composition of Hospital Infection Control Committees vary as do the patterns of attendance

Departmental Guidance Suggested membership	Number of NHS Trusts who specified membership	Always/ Sometimes attends[1]	Rarely /Never attends	Didn't answer
Chief Executive[2]	22 (11%)	14 (64%)	5 (23%)	3 (14%)
Chief Executive Representative[2]	138 (65%)	123 (90%)	6 (4%)	9 (7%)
CCDC	174 (81%)	156 (89%)	9 (6%)	9 (6%)
Infection Control Doctor	205 (96%)	190 (93%)	-	15 (7%)
Infection Control Nurse	209 (98%))	194 (93%)	-	15 (7%)
Occupational Health Physician[2]	126 (59)	98 (78%)	19 (15%)	9 (8%)
Occupational Health Nurse[2]	163 (76%)	151 (93%)	3 (2%)	9 (6%)
Infectious Disease Physician	38 (18%)	30 (79%)	6 (16%)	2 (6%)
Senior Clinical Medical Staff	182 (85%)	142 (78%)	25 (14%)	15 (8%)
Nurse Executive Director	132 (62%)	110 (84%)	8 (6%)	14 (11%)
Representative from other hospitals covered by HICC (n=120 NHS Trust)	62 (29%)	26 (42%)	6 (10%)	9 (15%)

Notes: 1. Not all respondents who answered membership question detailed frequency of attendance

2. Either / or both can be members

Source: National Audit Office census, analysis of the membership of the 215 trusts who stated that they had a Hospital Infection Control Committee

---

2.16 Seventy seven per cent of Hospital Infection Control Committees meet at least quarterly, ninety seven per cent produce minutes of their meetings (3 per cent didn't answer the question) but only 52 per cent produce an annual report. Sixty eight per cent sent their minutes to the chief executive, 87 per cent of those producing an annual report sent it to the chief executive.

In NHS Trusts with an infection control programme, the programme did not always comply with Departmental guidance

2.17 The Chief Executive's responsibility for ensuring that there are effective infection control arrangements includes the need to put an effective infection control programme with defined objectives in place[9]. We found that in 170 NHS Trusts (79 per cent) the infection control team had an infection control programme. In those NHS Trusts without a formal programme, we were told that infection control activities were either planned at the Hospital Infection Control Committee meetings or, in about half the cases, infection control activities were a reaction to problems and requests.

2.18 The Hospital Infection Control Committee is expected to discuss and endorse the infection control team's annual infection control programme which should then be submitted for approval to the chief executive (Departments 1995 guidance[9]). However, only 11 per cent of chief executives (19 NHS Trusts) told us that they personally formally approved the infection control programme with 75 per cent approved by the Hospital Infection Control Committee, (other NHS Trusts did not reply to this question). Approval by the Hospital Infection Control Committee may be appropriate in those NHS Trusts where the chief executive is a member and regularly attends the Committee (14 NHS Trusts). Nonetheless we are concerned that this may reduce the authority of the programme in these trusts where the chief executive neither personally approves the programme nor is party to its approval as a member of the Hospital Infection Control Committee.

2.19 Where NHS Trusts had infection control programmes our analysis showed generally high compliance with Departmental guidance on content (Figure 9). For example, 94 per cent of NHS Trusts complied with the need to produce, review and update infection control policies. However, compliance was lower in relation to standard setting and audit of the hospital's clinical and support services and setting standards for the infection control teams own activities with just over half of the programmes including these aspects. These are important parts of the cycle to improve infection control, and without them NHS Trusts cannot evaluate the effectiveness and the extent of the implementation of policies. Indeed it is important that all NHS Trusts should include all of the activities covered in Figure 9 in the programme as they have a direct bearing on the prevention, detection and control of hospital acquired infection.

Analysis of Content of NHS Trusts' 1997-98 Infection Control Programmes for planning infection control

Figure 9	

The majority of programmes included the production, review and monitoring of policies. 23 NHS Trusts did not include surveillance and over a third did not include audit or standard setting.

Recommended Activity	Number and percentage of NHS Trusts where activity was included in programme[1]	
	Number	%
Production, review and update of policies	163	94
Monitoring of hospital hygiene	153	88
Staff training and education	150	86
Planned surveillance activities	146	84
Input to standard setting and audit of clinical and support services	103	59
Audit of infection control team activities	90	52

Source: National Audit Office Census

Note: 1. The analysis is based on the 174 NHS Trusts who replied that they did have a programme.

Funding arrangements for infection control in hospitals are varied

2.20 The 1995 Departmental guidance[9] noted that NHS Trusts need to have flexibility in the use of their resources but there are advantages for the planning and implementation of an effective infection control programme if infection control teams have a separate budget for routine infection control work.

2.21 We found that some 40 per cent of infection control teams had a separate budget for control of infection in the hospital, but that the elements included within the separate budgets varied significantly. Few budgets included all of the elements suggested by Departmental guidance (Figure 10). For example less than a quarter of budgets included funding for infection control doctor's time and microbiology testing. These activities are funded out of other budgets within the NHS Trust.

Figure 10
Items included in NHS Trust infection control budgets

Budget elements recommended in Departmental guidance[2]	No of NHS Trusts including item in budget	% of NHS Trusts including item in budget[1]
Infection control doctor's time	17	20
Employment of infection control nurse(s)	76	89
Clerical and laboratory support staff costs	48	56
Microbiology tests and equipment specifically needed for infection control	18	21
Computer equipment for surveillance	25	29
Educational aids, videos, posters etc.	60	70
Training and education of infection control team members and provision of books, journals etc	63	74
Printing and dissemination of policies and manuals	45	53
Travel between institutions covered by infection control team	61	71

Notes: 1. There were 86 NHS Trusts (40%) with a separate budget for routine infection control.

2. The cost of managing outbreaks or other major infection incidents should be met from other sources such as contingency funds or insurance cover. If the infection control team provides infection control services outside the main hospital these should be the subject of a clearly defined contract with associated funding (Department's 1995 guidance[9]).

Source: National Audit Office census comparing actual contents against Departmental guidance

2.22 In NHS Trusts with a separate budget, the amounts allocated to the budget varied widely. One infection control team told us that the amount allocated to their budget in 1997-98 was £500, which covered the cost of publications only. At the other extreme, another infection control team had a budget of nearly £1 million, which included all of the elements specified in the Departmental guidance.

2.23 The lack of separate budgets, and the incomplete coverage of those that exist, means that many NHS Trusts cannot readily see how much infection control costs or make fully informed decisions on infection control spending. Of the infection control teams who did not have their own budget, 67 considered that their management of infection control would be improved if they had a separate infection control budget as it would facilitate better planning, prioritisation, control and flexibility. However, 16 infection control teams felt that it would hinder their management and 37 that it would make no difference.

Requirements to control infection in hospital may not be matched by resources to do it

2.24 When the Standards in Infection Control were introduced in 1993[14], the Department encouraged NHS Trusts to comply with the standards but did not provide any additional hypothecated funding. This was in line with the wider resource allocation policy in which Public Expenditure Survey allocations to health authorities were not generally earmarked for specific purposes. In 1995, when the Department's guidance was issued under cover of Health Service Guidelines HSG(95)10[9], this stated that the need to comply with the guidelines "should have no financial or manpower implications".

2.25 Because many infection control teams' resources, including staff, are allocated for budgetary purposes in other work units it is not possible to draw firm conclusions about relative changes in funding of infection control over time. However infection control teams reported to us that, in their opinion after allowing for salary increases, there has been little real term change in the funding of infection control in hospitals in the last three years (Figure 11). Our analysis shows that only 7 per cent of infection control teams considered that the amount of money budgeted for infection control had increased between 1996-97 and 1997-98 and again, only 7 per cent of infection control teams believed the budget had increased between 1997-98 and 1998-9. During this time, expectations, particularly in relation to a number of resource intensive activities including surveillance, have increased. Infection control teams told us that NHS Trust policies, like movement of patients between beds and between wards, quicker throughput of patients and greater use of invasive techniques are also increasing the demand on their time and resources. Overall, we believe that in many NHS Trusts there may be a growing mismatch between what is expected of infection control teams in controlling hospital infection and the resources allocated to them.

Change in funding of infection control over the last three years[1]

Figure 11

Change in infection control budget	Increased	Decreased	Stayed the same
Percentage change 1996/97 - 1997/98	15 (7%)	4 (2%)	197 (91%)
Percentage change 1997/98 – 1998/99	15 (7%)	8 (4%)	193 (89%)

Note: 1. The question asked was "In your opinion, apart from increases to meet annual increase in salaries, has the amount of money budgeted for infection control increased, decreased or stayed the same between 1996-97 and 1997-98 and 1997-98 and 1998-99, whether as a separate budget or generally?" The question did not ask staff to verify their answers with figures for those without a separate budget, so there is inevitably an element of perception as to how the amount of resources available might have changed.

Source: National Audit Office census

Staffing ratios for infection control work vary widely

2.26 The Department's 1995 guidance stressed that every hospital should have an infection control team comprising an infection control doctor and infection control nurse(s). This team has the primary responsibility for, and reports to the chief executive on, all aspects of surveillance, prevention and control of infection in the hospital. An important strategic issue is whether infection control teams have sufficient staff to deal with these requirements in their NHS Trust. A good measure of the demands on infection control staff is the number of beds in the NHS Trust, as this is related to throughput of patients and in turn to the potential number of cases of hospital acquired infections. There are no explicit Departmental guidelines for the ratio of the number of infection control nurses or infection control doctors to beds or the amount of time required for the various activities of consultant microbiologists, as NHS Trusts are expected to determine staffing levels based on assessment of size of the hospital, case mix, throughput and the need to provide 24 hour cover.[9]

2.27 Most infection control doctors are consultant medical microbiologists. In October 1997, in evidence to the House of Lords inquiry into Antibiotic Resistance[24] the Association of Medical Microbiologists stated that "the number of medical microbiologists has remained approximately constant or even fallen over the last few years while the workload of their laboratories has increased substantially". Using data generated from 49 hospital departments of microbiology (The Clinical Benchmarking Co, 1997) serious concerns were expressed about the inadequacy of numbers of microbiologists and the way this impacted unfavourably on infection control activities and thus the prevention of hospital acquired infection[24].

2.28 In the absence of Departmental guidelines for the time that infection control doctors should spend on infection control, in June 1999, the Royal College of Pathologists issued guidelines based on indicative assessments of the amount of time required for the various activities of consultant microbiologists[25]. In relation to infection control, they recommended that, in a 500 bed district general hospital, consultants should:

- spend a minimum of 3 sessions a week (10.5 hours) on infection control activities such as providing advice, chairing meetings, provision and revision of policies, investigating outbreaks, commissioning wards/theatres, educational activities etc;

■ spend 1-2 hours per day (5-10 per week) on interpreting laboratory results including the provision of advice on patient management (particularly antibiotic treatment and the need for isolation/barrier nursing) and any other investigations that may be needed. For specialist units such as Intensive Care, Transplant and Renal units etc. each unit will require a further one hour (this equates to between 2 and 3 sessions) per week; also

■ be part of a team providing a rota to fulfil the requirement for 24 hour cover.

2.29 For a 500 bed hospital with an average of 2 specialist units this would mean that between 5 and 6 sessions a week should be devoted to infection control. As a consultant's full time contract comprises 11 sessions a week, this is the equivalent to around 50 percent of the infection control doctors time, which should be spent on infection control duties. This would mean that there should be 1 Whole Time Equivalent (WTE) infection control doctor to 1000 beds. We found that only 46 infection control teams met this ratio. The mean staffing ratio was 1: 2,258 beds and the median 1:1,817 beds (Figure 12).

2.30 In most NHS Trusts infection control doctors told us that their numbers had stayed relatively static during the last three years. For example 176 infection control teams (81 per cent) told us that their resources had stayed the same, 23 (11 per cent) that they had increased and 10 (5 per cent) that they had decreased. Ten infection control teams told us that they had difficulty recruiting an infection control doctor and two that they had a vacancy for more than 13 months, mainly due to specific local shortages. Some Trusts have adopted different staffing models for infection control. For example, managers and clinicians at the Hammersmith Hospitals Trust made a successful business case to the Trust to provide additional resources for infection control activities (Case Study 3).

Case Study 3

A new development in infection control and hospital epidemiology at Hammersmith Hospitals Trust integrated into an Academic Department of Infectious Diseases and Microbiology

Problem

Managers and clinicians at Hammersmith Hospital recognised that infection control was an issue of growing importance with significant resource implications, and could not be properly addressed by the existing complement of medical microbiologists who were already heavily committed.

Solution

They therefore made a successful business case to the Trust to provide additional resources for infection control activities, to include funding for a new consultant position, together with appropriate support for data management and secretarial help. In parallel, the Academic Department of Infectious Diseases at Imperial College contributed part of the consultant salary, thus allowing the appointment of the first Senior Lecturer in Infection Control and Hospital Epidemiology in the UK.

Outcome

The Senior Lecturer works within the broader department of Infectious Disease and Microbiology and so has close clinical and academic contacts with relevant colleagues. This innovative approach which has provided a consultant-level appointment dealing exclusively with infection control issues has already resulted in a more proactive approach to infection control within the Trust, as well as highlighting some problems which had not been fully appreciated. It should also provide a focus for academic and educational initiatives in this field.

Figure 12

The ratio of whole time equivalent infection control doctors to total number of beds in NHS Trusts

There is a wide variation in the ratio of infection control doctors to beds in NHS Trusts.

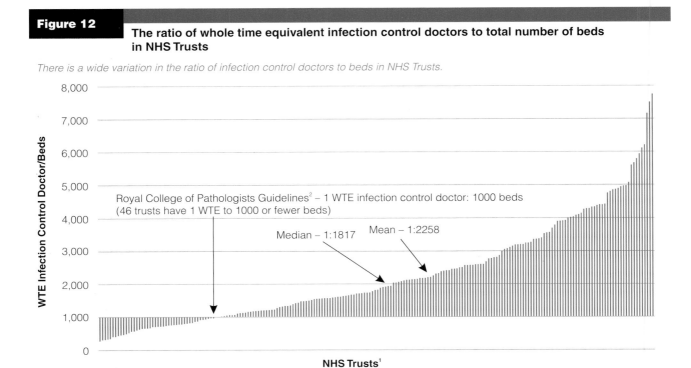

Notes:
1. Excludes 8 trusts who either have no infection control doctor, with infection control doctor role being provided by a neighbouring trust, and 4 who have very low ICD to bed ratio.

2. Guideline is that an ICD in a 500 bed DGH should spend 3 sessions (10.5 hr) devoted to infection control activities such as: monitoring; investigating outbreaks; supporting occupational health departments; commissioning wards and theatres; kitchen inspections; education activities; provision of advice on patient management. This approximates to a Total of 5.5 sessions for the average 500 bed DGH or 50% of 1 WTE ICD.

Source: National Audit Office census

There are wide variations in the ratio of infection control nurses to beds in NHS Trusts

2.31 In the early 1970s a number of American studies recommended that there should be one infection control nurse to every 250 beds. The comprehensive SENIC study (Haley et al)[8] strongly supported the 250 bed recommendation. The study concluded "essential components of effective programs included conducting organised surveillance and having a trained, effectual infection control physician, an infection control nurse per 250 beds, and a system for reporting infection rates to practising surgeons. Programs with these components reduced their hospitals infection rates by 32 per cent". Subsequently the ratio of 1/250 was adopted as a requirement for accreditation from the Joint Committee for Accreditation of Healthcare Organisations. We found that in the absence of any guidelines or benchmarks the 1/250 is widely quoted by English NHS Trusts in business cases requesting additional staff resources.

2.32 From our survey of infection control team staffing we found a wide variation in the ratio of infection control nurses to beds (Figure 13). The average ratio of infection control nurses' time (in whole time equivalents) to beds in NHS Trusts is one infection control nurse to 535 beds (the median is 1: 472). Eighty seven per cent of NHS Trusts had ratios that were higher than the 1: 250 figure. Two NHS Trusts did not have any infection control nurses in post at the time of our survey. Overall, we consider that in some NHS Trusts, particularly those in the top quartile of the distribution, the number of beds that a single infection control nurse is expected to cover is unacceptably high. However, the Department does not believe that in the absence of explicit guidelines this conclusion can be drawn (Figure 13).

2.33 In 123 (57 per cent) of NHS Trusts, the whole time equivalent number of infection control nurses has stayed the same over the last three years. Over the same period, 67 infection control teams (31 per cent) have experienced an increase in their nursing complement and 20 (9 per cent) have experienced a decrease. Twenty four teams told us that they had had difficulties recruiting infection control nurses with nine teams carrying a vacancy for more than seven months. Sixty infection control teams told us that they had prepared a business case for extra infection control nurse resources: 24 of these were successful, 16 were unsuccessful and the decision is unknown or pending on a further 20 cases. Case Study 4 shows a successful business case.

2.34 We are concerned that the wide variations in resources for both infection control nurses and doctors may represent unacceptable differences that could impact on the quality of care that patients can expect regarding hospital acquired infection and infection control generally in hospital. Parts 3 and 4 consider among other things, the availability of resources and how this impacts on the infection control teams ability to carry out their infection control prevention, detection and control activities. We consider that all trusts should evaluate their infection control arrangements to determine whether their infection control function is adequately resourced.

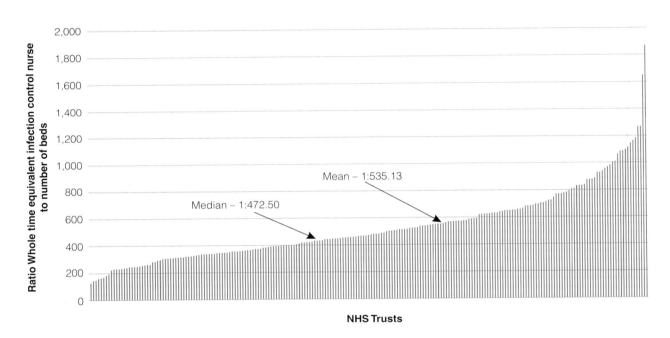

Figure 13

The Ratio of whole time equivalent infection control nurses to total number of beds in NHS Trusts

There is a wide variation in the ratio of infection control nurse time to beds in NHS Trusts.

Ratio Whole time equivalent infection control nurse to number of beds

Mean – 1:535.13

Median – 1:472.50

NHS Trusts

Sample Size: 218 NHS Trusts

Source: National Audit Office Census

Case Study 4

A good case can be made for increasing Infection Control Team resources - Guy's and St Thomas NHS Trust

Problem   An audit of the infection control arrangements at Guy's and St Thomas's NHS Trust revealed a high infection control staff workload and conditions associated with a an increased risk of hospital infection. These included high levels of agency staff, a significant lack of simple facilities such as handwash basins and relatively few isolation facilities. The audit identified that further increases in infection control workload would be necessary if the NHS Trust was to comply with Departmental guidelines. They identified a need for a further 2 infection control nurses to undertake this workload.

Solution   The Infection Control Team put forward a business case to the NHS Trust Board. This indicated that the estimated annual cost of hospital acquired infection was £3.9m (based on the number of admissions, an extra length of stay of three days and an average cost of 1 bed day of £200).

However, with an efficient infection control programme and resources to undertake it, the Infection Control Team estimated that cost savings of at least £1million per annum could be achieved. There would be increased patient throughput, reduced waiting lists and reduced unit costs of patient admissions.

Outcome   The business case was successful and the NHS Trust agreed funding for 2 extra Infection Control Nurses.

Some NHS Trusts use link nurses

2.35   Link nurses are not substitutes for Infection Control Nurses but are ward based staff who act under the supervision of the Infection Control Nurse. They should have sufficient clinical experience and standing to have authority with managers and colleagues. Their aim is to help increase awareness of infection control issues and assist in the early detection of infection outbreaks. In some cases they have been trained to collect surveillance data for the infection control team.

2.36   We found that 128 NHS Trusts (59 per cent) use the link nurse system, of which 18 per cent considered it to be fairly unsuccessful or not successful at all. Another 16 NHS Trusts (7 per cent) have tried the link nurse system and abandoned it because of high staff turnover and because wards nominated junior nurses to act as link nurses but they lacked authority with other members of staff.

At least half of the 128 NHS Trusts who used link nurses reported that they found that it was fairly successful in improving infection control, particularly in terms of improving awareness, and a fifth thought it was very successful. Link nurses might not be appropriate for all NHS Trusts, particularly large NHS Trusts with multiple sites and high staff turnover. They are effective when: there is a relatively stable workforce; the hospital is on a small number of sites; the nurses have recognised authority; and they are allocated time to attend meetings and training sessions. Case Study 5 gives an example of a successful link nurse programme in one NHS Trust.

Most infection control teams believe that they have inadequate clerical support

2.37 Infection control doctors and nurses need adequate clerical and secretarial support so that they can concentrate on prevention and control activities. We found that the availability of clerical support was very varied. Twenty seven per cent of infection control teams (59 teams) had no support and just over half of the infection control teams had less than one whole time equivalent. Overall, 63 per cent of infection control doctors and 70 per cent of infection control nurses considered that clerical support was inadequate. As a result they considered that they spent a disproportionate amount of their own time on administrative and clerical activities, leaving less time for surveillance, prevention and control activities. The Department pointed out that the infection control teams view about the lack of clerical support is not a surprising finding since many NHS professionals feel that they could function more effectively if they had more support staff.

Case Study 5

The development of an Infection Control link nurse programme at the Mid Essex Hospital Services NHS Trust

Problem

The Infection Control Team were concerned that the profile of infection control was not particularly high, with responsibility placed solely on one Infection Control Doctor and one Infection Control Nurse in a 860 bed NHS Trust. The Infection Control Team convinced the NHS Trust that better infection control and feedback to clinicians could reduce infection rates and save costs.

Solution

The NHS Trust therefore agreed to develop an Infection Control link nurse programme, which would be introduced over 4 years in 3 phases: setting up and establishing; ward standard setting; and management ownership. Each ward and department was asked to nominate a link nurse and deputy, who became part of the Infection Control Liaison Group - a total of 57 link nurses. These nurses are readily identifiable to ward staff and have regular contact with the Infection Control Team including 3-monthly formal training sessions. Their main responsibilities are education and surveillance. The NHS Trust has recognised the importance of link nurses by awarding them formal contracts.

Outcome

The link nurse programme has raised the profile of infection control. The Infection Control Team has been incorporated into the risk management group at NHS Trust level giving infection control a high status and authority. Their knowledge base and the reliability and coverage of surveillance has increased significantly and there is evidence that infection rates and costs due to hospital acquired infection have reduced.

Source: Synopsis of Article submitted in response to our census and also published in the Journal of Hospital Infection (1996)34, 167-278

Infection control teams report a lack of IT necessary to do their job effectively

2.38 The Infection Control Nurses Association in their evidence to the House of Lords Select Committee on Science and Technology[24] emphasised that the infection control team is much more effective when they have resources in terms of clerical staff and information technology but that few had access to either resource. The Committee drew particular attention to the scope for IT to facilitate surveillance of disease and antibiotic resistance. Infection Control Teams told us that lack of computer hardware and software was a major constraint to carrying out their infection control duties effectively. We found that over half of infection control teams did not have their own computer or access to one for recording and analysing data, especially surveillance information, or for producing reports to clinicians and nurses.

2.39 Only 40 per cent of infection control doctors have access to other NHS Trust information systems for identifying patients who have been readmitted to hospital with an infection, and who may be a source of hospital acquired infections. Very few infection control doctors and infection control nurses have access to pharmacy prescribing data, which makes aspects of infection control work such as monitoring antibiotic policies difficult.

2.40 Of those who had their own computerised systems, few were able to download information automatically and had to enter data manually. This takes up time which could be spent more productively. Also, surveillance work is made more time consuming and difficult if case details have to be obtained from case notes, rather than from computerised information systems.

2.41 The NHS Executive's action plan for the NHS (HSG 1999/049),[20] acknowledged the problems caused by lack of appropriate IT. It highlighted the need to ensure that the implementation of the new NHS Information Strategy supports the information needs for the prevention and control of communicable disease and infection, including that caused by antimicrobial resistant organisms. For NHS Trusts, the Information for Health Strategy[26] expects 35% of NHS Trusts to have installed electronic patient record systems (including reporting results of prescribing) by 2002, and all NHS Trusts by 2005.

There is scope to use the development of controls assurance to improve NHS Trusts' approach to hospital acquired infection

2.42 Controls assurance is a process whereby Trust Boards can assure the public that the Trust operates an effective system of internal control covering key risks. Chief executives of NHS Trusts and health authorities are currently required to sign a controls assurance statement in respect of the system of internal financial controls in their annual accounts. From November 1999, this requirement has been extended to wider non-financial, non-clinical risk by the production of controls assurance statements to accompany the annual report.[21] By 31 March 2000 NHS Trusts and health authorities are required to have completed a baseline self assessment against the published risk management and organisational standards. They are then expected to produce statements setting out their plans to implement the requirements by July 2000.

2.43 The standards for infection control include management structures and responsibilities, policies and procedures, education and training, surveillance and microbiological services. Verification of standards is likely to be carried out by internal audit, with specialist training given to internal auditors to enable them to work with relevant technical specialists. Work is underway to identify the nature and extent of any external review and verification activity beyond 1999-2000. The expectation is that national performance assessments will be carried out by the Commission for Health Improvement and the Audit Commission. These developments should help clarify the accountability mechanisms and help to improve the overall approach to hospital acquired infection within each NHS Trust.

Improving strategic management of hospital acquired infection

2.44 A number of NHS Trusts have put infection control high on their agenda and there are also a number of good practice examples where infection control teams have made efforts to overcome staffing and other resource constraints. The Department's positive response to the House of Lords Select Committee inquiry[18] should go some way towards improving the strategic management of hospital acquired infection, as should their new infection control standards issued as part of control assurance in the NHS.[21] However, we have identified areas where NHS Trusts can improve the strategic management of infection control still further. In particular:

The Department should:

- consider the need for a revision of their 1995 guidance on infection control and ensure that the implementation of the controls assurance standard on infection control is monitored through the NHS performance management process and through the Commission for Health Improvement and the Audit Commission;

- consider commissioning research on appropriate staffing levels for the infection control team, to help NHS Trusts determine an appropriate level of resources; and

- ensure necessary access to any relevant systems developed as part of its NHS Information Management and Technology Strategy.

Health authorities and NHS Trusts need to work together (and in the future with Primary Care Groups and Trusts) to:

■ review their service agreements, with input from the Consultant in Communicable Disease Control and infection control team to ensure that each NHS Trust's arrangements meet recently issued controls assurance standards on hospital acquired infection; and

■ ensure that service agreements require the collection of data on the rates and trends of hospital acquired infection, based on surveillance.

Chief executives of NHS Trusts need to ensure that:

■ the infection control team has an adequate annual programme for infection control that is approved by them and that they and the Trust Board receive regular feedback on performance in relation to the strategy and programme; and

■ as part of the requirement to put infection control and basic hygiene at the heart of good management and clinical practice:

a) their senior management and clinicians are encouraged to accept greater ownership for the control of hospital acquired infection;

b) the Hospital Infection Control Committee is operating as the Department intended and that they or their nominated deputy attends meetings;

c) the infection control function is resourced in line with Departmental guidance; and

d) in developing their IT systems as part of the Information Strategy for the Modern NHS 1998-2005, their action plan takes into account the requirements of the infection control team, particularly in relation to surveillance.

Part 3: Surveillance and its effectiveness in reducing hospital acquired infection

3.1 Hospital acquired infection can have serious consequences for patients and may be costing the NHS as much as £1 billion a year[12]. While it is acknowledged that there will be an irreducible minimum, it is important that all reasonable steps are taken to reduce the extent of avoidable hospital acquired infection within individual NHS Trusts. This part of the report considers the extent to which hospital acquired infection is realistically preventable and the effectiveness of surveillance as a key infection control measure.

Most infection control teams believe that between 5 and 20 per cent of hospital acquired infection is preventable

3.2 In 1995, the Department stated in its guidance[9] that "overall we believe that about 30 per cent of hospital acquired infection could be prevented by better application of existing knowledge and implementation of realistic infection control policies". We asked infection control teams whether they considered this level of prevention could be achieved in their NHS Trust. Eighty five infection control teams (39 per cent) considered that it could be, 106 (49 per cent) felt that the 30 per cent figure was too high and 12 per cent either did not know or did not answer the question.

3.3 We asked infection control teams to estimate the level of infection which, in their view, was preventable in their Trust and obtained a wide range of responses (Figure 14). The most common estimate (from about a fifth of infection control teams who responded) was that a reduction of between 5 and 10 per cent in hospital acquired infection is possible. However, a similar number felt the scope for reduction was higher (18 per cent of infection control teams thought a reduction of between 11 and 15 per cent was possible and 14 per cent that a reduction of between 16 and 20 per cent was possible). The bed weighted average across all NHS Trusts that provided an estimate was 15 per cent.

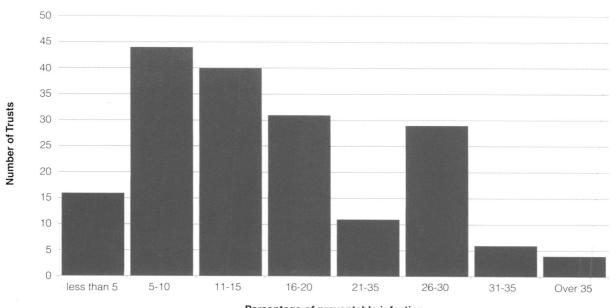

Figure 14

Distribution of infection control teams views on the percentage of hospital acquired infection that is preventable in their NHS Trust

Percentage of preventable infection

Note: This figure, which is based on the 174 infection control teams who answered the question, shows grouped responses from infection control teams without allowing for their size of their individual Trust. Calculating a bed weighted average from the responses, indicates that 15 per cent of hospital acquired infection could be prevented.

Source: National Audit Office census

Reducing hospital acquired infection would bring significant patient benefits and avoidable costs could be as much as £150 million per annum

3.4 Attributing costs to a hospital acquired infection is complex and uncertain. The recent study by the London School of Hygiene and Tropical Medicine and the Public Health Laboratory Service[12], commissioned by the Department of Health, provides the most recent estimate. This estimate, which is derived from a comprehensive and detailed review of the cost of infection in one hospital, suggests that hospital acquired infection may cost the NHS in England almost £1 billion a year. On this basis, the potentially avoidable level of hospital acquired infections imposes a cost of £150 million a year. This is inevitably a broad-brush estimate as it depends on extrapolating data from one hospital across the NHS, assumes that achievable reductions are across the full range of infections and does not allow for the cost of measures that would be needed to achieve reductions in hospital acquired infection. While there are few published reports on reliable UK trials of cost effective prevention measures, we regard the figure of £150 million a year as a useful indicator of the possible gross savings that could be made.

3.5 The London School of Hygiene and Tropical Medicine and Public Health Laboratory Service study team recommend that further work is needed to determine the cost effectiveness of selected infection control practices. They acknowledge that although their results provide important information on the magnitude and distribution of costs incurred by patients who acquire an infection in hospital they do not directly inform decisions about allocation of resources. While we endorse their recommendations we consider that, in the meantime, individual NHS Trusts need to identify the main risks to patients of hospital acquired infection and target their infection control resources accordingly.

Effective surveillance is essential to reduce hospital infection rates and associated costs

3.6 Surveillance is an essential component of the prevention and control of infection in hospitals. It consists of the routine collection of data on infections among patients and staff, its analysis and dissemination of results to those who need to know so that appropriate action can be taken. The main objectives of surveillance are:

■ the prevention and early detection of outbreaks in order to allow timely investigation and control;

■ the assessment of infection levels over time in order to determine the need for, and measure the effect of, preventative or control measures.

3.7 In response to our survey, a large proportion of infection control doctors and infection control nurses stated that they would like to spend less time on being reactive and more time on surveillance in order to reduce hospital acquired infection. Evidence given to the House of Lords Select Committee on Science and Technology enquiry on Antibiotic Resistance[10] made the same point.

3.8 Infection control teams are supported in their wish to spend more time on surveillance by evidence from a comprehensive five year study of infection control in over 300 hospitals in the United States of America (the SENIC project - Haley et al, 1985).[8] This showed that hospitals with infection control programmes which included surveillance and feedback to clinicians reduced infections by an average of 32 per cent. In contrast, hospitals with an infection control programme that excluded surveillance reduced rates by 6 per cent over five years, and those without effective programmes saw rates increase by 18 per cent. The research concluded that without organised routine surveillance systems, even the most rigorous infection control policies are unlikely to be fully successful.

Departmental guidance recommends a strategy for surveillance

3.9 The Department's 1995 guidance[9] details examples of various methods of surveillance together with the advantages and disadvantages of each method. The guidance also draws attention to the work of one study, Glenister et al[5] in 1992, which was commissioned by the Department to compare selective surveillance methods over an extended period of time against a comprehensive standard method designed to detect all infections in the population being studied. This study identified the best general method as laboratory based ward liaison surveillance, involving follow up of positive microbiology reports with review of patients case records plus twice weekly visits to the wards to review patients considered by ward staff to have an infection.

3.10 Based on these conclusions, the 1995 guidance recommended that the infection control team, together with the Hospital Infection Control Committee, should develop a surveillance strategy, based on:

■ continuous "alert" organism surveillance, which uses laboratory reports to identify specific organisms, and "alert" condition surveillance, in which ward staff have a responsibility to report specific clinical conditions to the infection control team. These surveillance methods should cover the whole Trust with the results being reported to the infection control team on a daily basis;

■ pro-active continuous surveillance of microbiology specimens and laboratory results from the whole hospital to detect outbreaks or other unexpected changes in patterns of all types of infection. This requires the infection control team to scrutinise positive microbiology results on a daily basis: for example, blood cultures; cerebrospinal fluid; catheters removed from infected intravenous sites; samples from intensive care units; post-operative wound swabs; and urine samples; and

3.16 In 1995, following a competitive tendering exercise, the Department commissioned a project to develop a national surveillance scheme. The project, which was awarded to the Public Health Laboratory Service in November 1995, is managed jointly by the Department and Public Health Laboratory Service. The aims of this Nosocomial (meaning hospital acquired) Infection National Surveillance Scheme are:

■ to improve patient care by assisting hospitals to change clinical practice and reduce rates and risk of hospital acquired infection; and

■ to provide national statistics on hospital acquired infection for comparison with local results.

3.17 The scheme was launched in March 1996 with around 30 hospitals taking part in a pilot phase. This was then carried forward until March 2000, with a total budget of £2.5 million, half of which was provided by the Department. The aim was that ultimately most acute hospitals would eventually participate in the Nosocomial Infection National Surveillance Scheme.

Many NHS Trusts have obtained benefits from their participation, but various problems need to be overcome for the scheme to be fully effective

3.18 We consider that the Nosocomial Infection National Surveillance Scheme is an important infection control tool because it:

■ allows participating NHS Trusts to judge their performance against data from comparable patient groups in other hospitals;

■ enables participating NHS Trusts to work with the Nosocomial Infection National Surveillance Scheme team and others to use the results to try and make any improvements that appear to be needed;

■ has the potential to develop into a truly national scheme with the scope to produce year on year data that will allow trends in hospital acquired infection in England to be monitored; and

■ offers scope to adapt the methodology and results for use as a quality assessment tool, as part fulfilment of the requirements of the NHS Clinical Governance initiative[19].

3.19 At the time of our survey, 31 NHS Trusts told us that they had participated in the pilot scheme and 94 NHS Trusts that they had or were participating in one or both modules of the Nosocomial Infection National Surveillance Scheme (relating to surgical site infections and hospital acquired bacteraemia (bloodstream) infection). Forty two per cent of these NHS Trusts said they had experienced benefits, while 44 per cent believe that they had not as yet seen the benefits. The remaining NHS Trusts did not answer the question. Figure 17 summarises the main benefits and problems experienced by participating NHS Trusts. We asked these Trusts whether, given it is still early in the life of the scheme, they had experienced any benefits from their participation. The main benefits were the standardisation of data collection and the ability to compare results and the main problems were the time needed to collect data and the general strain on resources imposed by surveillance.

Some of the benefits and problems experienced by infection control teams participating in the Nosocomial Infection National Surveillance Scheme

Figure 17

Some of the main benefits cited by infection control teams were:

■ the ability to compare results and trends within and between NHS Trusts (12 Trusts);

■ that it raised the profile and increased awareness of the importance of infection control (12 NHS Trusts);

■ that it provided a structured approach to data collection and analysis (8 NHS Trusts); and

■ that it introduced clinical and medical staff to the concept of independent surveillance and objective data collection (12 NHS Trusts).

Over the next 2-3 years the expected benefits of participation included:

■ that good aggregate data would facilitate performance evaluation which avoided the league table type of assessment (32 NHS Trusts); and

■ that it should lead to a general reduction by managing rates and risks (8 NHS Trusts); and

■ the ability to use the results to identify areas of concern (3 NHS Trusts), apply for greater resources (3 NHS Trusts) and influence contracts with health authorities (2 NHS Trusts).

Teams that believed they had not as yet experienced any benefits cited the following problems:

■ the time needed to collect data made data collection problematic (39 NHS Trusts);

■ surveillance was a strain on resources (19 NHS Trusts);

■ feedback of results was too slow (16 NHS Trusts) and difficult to understand (2 NHS Trusts);

■ the reports on the results were difficult to interpret (7 NHS Trusts);

■ teams lacked the necessary data collection tools, including IT (8 NHS Trusts); and

■ poor quality medical and nursing notes (5 NHS Trusts) and lack of co-operation from other NHS Trust staff constrained surveillance (3 NHS Trusts).

Source: National Audit Office census

Note: Some NHS Trusts gave several answers to the questions

3.20 On balance, NHS Trusts saw the Nosocomial Infection National Surveillance Scheme as a helpful innovation, and the number of hospitals who have participated has grown to 139 as at December 1999 (Figure 18), with a further 37 registering interest. New modules are currently under development for the surveillance of urinary tract infections and intensive care units.

The number of hospitals who have participated in one or more surveillance modules of the NINSS as at December 1999

Figure 18

The total number of hospitals which assisted with the pilot studies or participated in one or more module of NINSS as at 31 December 1999 was 139.

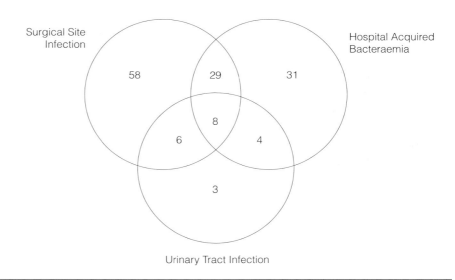

Surgical Site Infection

Hospital Acquired Bacteraemia

Urinary Tract Infection

58 29 31

8

6 4

3

Source: PHLS and Department of Health

The first year results from Nosocomial Infection National Surveillance Scheme suggest that there is scope to reduce hospital acquired infection

3.21 A report of the first year surveillance of surgical site infections, was published in December 1999.[16] A report on the surveillance of the first two years bacteraemia results is expected to be published soon. Although there are some limitations to the Nosocomial Infection National Surveillance Scheme data, namely the fact that it comprises self-selected hospitals, the first years data provides the most comprehensive set of comparable data available to the NHS. These data show variations between hospitals:

■ bacteraemia rates (May 1997 -April 1998) varied from 8.8 per 1000 patient days in General Intensive Care Units, to 5.3 for haematology patients and 0.3 for geriatric medicine; and

■ the average surgical wound infection per 100 operations for large bowel surgery was 10.6, compared with 2.5 per 100 total hip replacement operations and 1.9 for abdominal hysterectomies.

3.22 The reports show that there is generally scope to reduce hospital acquired infection. Also, that there may be some hospitals that can make large improvements (see Figures 19 and 20). While there may be valid reasons why a particular hospital is an outlier, this type of analysis allows the infection control team to investigate those reasons and to work with other NHS Trust staff to reduce the overall extent of hospital acquired infection.

Figure 19

Incidence of Hospital-acquired bacteraemia in participating hospitals medical specialties (data collection May 1997 to April 1998)

For all medical specialties the incidence of hospital acquired bacteraemia varied between hospitals. The range was particularly wide in haematology and oncology.

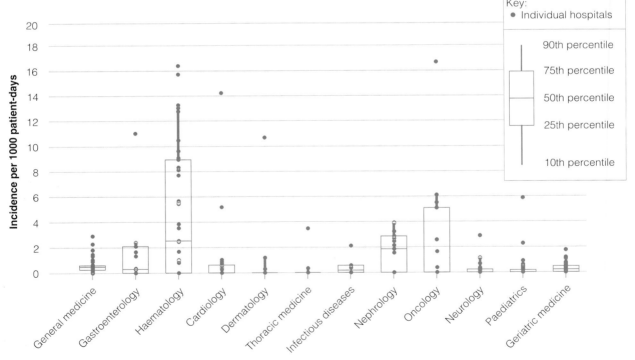

Note: Each point in the figure represents the incidence of hospital acquired bacteraemia for a participating hospital. Boxes placed on the sets of points for each category give the estimate of the 25th, 50th and 75th percentile and the ends of the vertical lines the 10th and 90th percentile.

Source: Central Public Health Laboratory Nosocomial Infection Surveillance Unit

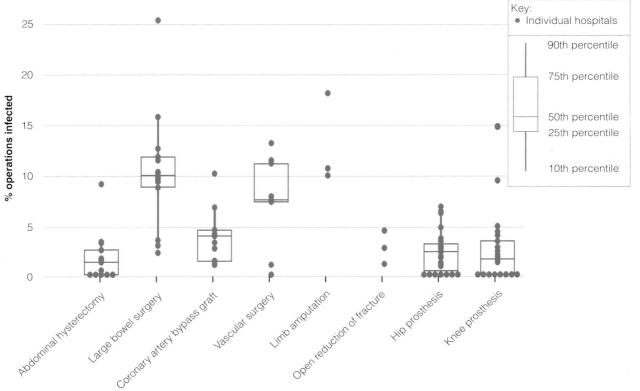

Figure 20

Distribution of the incidence of surgical site infection by category of surgical procedures (data collection October 1997 to September 1998)

For all surgical categories the incidence of surgical site infections varied between hospitals. The range was particularly wide in large bowel surgery.

Note: Each point in the figure represents the incidence of surgical site infection for a participating hospital. Boxes placed on the sets of points for each category give the estimates of the 25th, 50th and 75th percentiles of the incidence of surgical site infection and the ends of the vertical lines the 10th and 90th percentile.

Source: Central Public Health Laboratory Nosocomial Infection Surveillance Unit[16]

3.23 In order to realise these improvements in hospital acquired infection, clinicians need to be convinced of the merits of the Nosocomial Infection National Surveillance Scheme. One way of achieving this, and of overcoming the constraint of the infection control teams' perceived lack of resources to undertake surveillance, may be to give clinicians responsibility for surveillance, with the infection control team helping to facilitate data collection. In particular, surgeons should take responsibility for their own data on surgical site infections. Some NHS Trusts are exploring the use of staff outside the infection control team to collect data. In these NHS Trusts, the infection control team monitors the collection and undertakes analysis, interpretation and feedback of results, working with the clinicians to improve infection control.

There is inadequate feedback of Nosocomial Infection National Surveillance Scheme results within some NHS Trusts

3.24 Feedback of results is essential if NHS Trusts are to benefit from taking part in the Nosocomial Infection National Surveillance Scheme. In January 1999, the Nosocomial Infection National Surveillance Scheme team found that despite infection control teams having received the first year results of the bacteraemia module in November 1998, only a small proportion of Consultants in Communicable Disease Control, and only a handful of Hospital Infection Control Committees, had seen them. There was also evidence that NHS Trusts were not always feeding the Nosocomial Infection National Surveillance Scheme results back to the relevant clinicians. This limits the effectiveness of surveillance and may mean that action that should be taken to reduce hospital acquired infection is not being taken.

Appropriate software and additional training of surveillance personnel could overcome problems experienced by Nosocomial Infection National Surveillance Scheme

3.25 The equivalent of the Nosocomial National Surveillance Scheme, in the United States, is the National Nosocomial Infection Surveillance System. The American scheme has been operating for more than 30 years. It has grown from 19 participating hospitals to 230 and evolved from hospital wide surveillance to targeted surveillance. While 230 is still only a small proportion of the total number of hospitals in the United States, and a number of these are very small in comparison to English hospital Trusts, there are lessons from the scheme that may be applicable to the English scheme. For example, it uses customised computer software that facilitates the collection of information about rates of hospital acquired infection, and analysis of results by infection control teams and feedback of results to clinicians and senior management. The system also provides training in the use of the software.

3.26 The administrators of the American system, the National Center for Infectious Diseases (Centers for Disease Control) in Atlanta, told us that the software and training ensured accurate data with minimal need for cleaning which increased the efficiency and effectiveness of surveillance and facilitated prompt and accurate feedback. A 1996 paper in the Journal on Quality Improvement reviewed the "CDC Experience"[27] and gave examples of how the National Nosocomial Infection Surveillance System has been used as a tool for improving quality of care through the prevention of nosocomial infections. We believe that the approach adopted by the American scheme offers useful lessons for the Nosocomial Infection National Surveillance Scheme albeit the American system is operating in a different environment.

Nosocomial Infection National Surveillance Scheme could be extended to include information on antibiotic prescribing and antibiotic resistance

3.27 In England, the current Nosocomial Infection National Surveillance Scheme reports already provide some valuable information on antibiotic resistance in hospital acquired infection, for example the surgical site infections caused by MRSA as a proportion of all staphylococcal infections (Figure 21). This type of analysis provides a much needed overview of the situation with regard to antibiotic resistant organisms in participating hospitals and adds weight to the need for all acute hospitals to participate in the Nosocomial Infection National Surveillance Scheme.

3.28 The Public Health Laboratory Service is also developing a national Antibiotic Resistance Surveillance Programme that will provide comparative data on resistance, including resistance in hospital acquired infections at local, regional and national levels and will link these data to patterns of prescribing in hospitals and primary care. The first results of the pilot phase in the Trent region were reported to the Public Health Laboratory Service in December 1999.

3.29 The American system is being developed to enable information on antibiotic prescribing in intensive care units to be combined with data on infection rates so that changes in antibiotic resistance strains can be monitored. The House of Lords Inquiry on Antibiotic Resistance[10] recommended that the NHS should consider setting up something similar to the American research project in the UK, and the Department and Public Health Laboratory Service are currently considering whether a similar development could be incorporated into the Nosocomial Infection National Surveillance Scheme programme. As this will improve still further the value of national surveillance we fully endorse this development.

Figure 21

Distribution of micro-organisms identified as causing surgical site infections for all categories of surgical procedures

Almost half of the micro-organisms identified as causing infections were staphylococci, of which the majority were Staphylococcus aureus. Methicillin resistant staphylococcus aureus was the most common staphylococcus identified as causing surgical site infection in large bowel surgery, vascular surgery, limb amputation, open reduction of long bone fracture and bileduct, liver and pancreatic surgery.

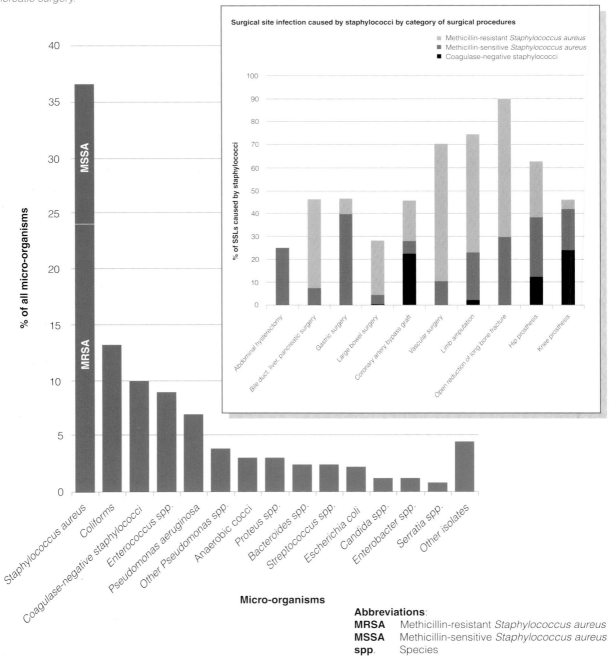

Micro-organisms

Abbreviations:
MRSA Methicillin-resistant *Staphylococcus aureus*
MSSA Methicillin-sensitive *Staphylococcus aureus*
spp. Species

Source: Central Public Health Laboratory Nosocomial Infection Surveillance Unit[16]

Future development of the National Infection National Surveillance Scheme

3.30 The Department has commissioned a review to determine the best ways to expand and develop the scheme to meet local NHS Trust and overall surveillance needs. As the current funding agreement expires on 31 March 2000 it is important that this review is concluded and future arrangements settled, as soon as possible.

Post discharge surveillance is important if NHS Trusts are to understand the full extent of hospital acquired infection but coverage to date has been patchy

3.31 The preceding paragraphs demonstrate that an increasing amount of effort is being spent on surveillance of hospital acquired infection. However, to date less attention has been given to post discharge surveillance. The main reason for this is the difficulty in determining an acceptable methodology and collecting comprehensive, reliable data. We found that post-discharge surveillance to monitor the extent that infections occur after discharge from hospital had been attempted in only a quarter of NHS Trusts. The most commonly used method was to provide the patient with a card/questionnaire to return if an infection occurred.

3.32 In recognition of the need for effective post-discharge surveillance the Department funded a Public Health Laboratory Service research study to evaluate post-discharge surveillance methods for surgical wound infection. Phase 1 was completed in 1997 and Phase 2 was planned to run from September 1998 to December 1999. The patients recruited into the study were from a wide range of surgical specialties, including day cases in three NHS Trusts. While it is acknowledged that identifying post discharge infections is not an exact science, the researchers believe that the methodology is robust for the majority of surgical specialties included in the study. The work shows that it is possible to collect data about post-discharge surveillance using patient reporting augmented by health care professional reporting.

3.33 Several studies have indicated that between 50 and 70 per cent of surgical wound infections occur post-discharge[7]. The preliminary findings from the Public Health Laboratory Service study would appear to support these findings. Some of the patients with post-discharge infections will have needed treatment from their general practitioners while others may have needed to be readmitted to hospital, both at a cost to the NHS. In addition most of these infections will have caused the patient additional discomfort. While we recognise that there is inevitably an element of uncertainty in determining whether an infection which manifests in the community necessarily implies a pre-discharge cause, the methodology developed by the study team appears robust. Without such information on post-discharge infection rates NHS Trusts are likely to be underestimating their performance in relation to hospital acquired infection. We therefore recommend that NHS Trusts should consider the need for some form of post-discharge surveillance, based on the methodology developed by the study team, either as part of the Nosocomial Infection National Surveillance Scheme or as part of NHS Trusts' own surveillance.

NHS Trusts have to balance the need to reduce hospital acquired infection against other key objectives

3.34 Preventing infection can be adversely affected by other NHS Trust-wide policies, especially bed management practice. Some infection control teams reported that the NHS drive to reduce waiting list levels has resulted in considerable pressure to achieve higher bed occupancy, and this is not always consistent with NHS Trust isolation, hygiene and cleaning practices, which are important means of reducing hospital acquired infection. Other developments such as placing beds close together, "hot-bedding", and patients moving frequently around the hospital as beds become free, can increase the risk of infection spreading.

3.35 The House of Lords Report[10] reported that "The Minister for Health conceded that faster throughput increases risk but is not incompatible with good practice." This is because faster throughput can itself lead to fewer hospital acquired infections if done in the interests of reducing the overall length of patients stay. The report went on to note that "A concomitant of general staff shortages and the pressures created by high bed occupancy is increasing reliance on agency nurses. Agency staff are sometimes poorly versed in infection control and may be unfamiliar with local procedures and, in moving frequently from one place of work to another, they may act as carriers of infection".

3.36 Should patients acquire an infection, their extended length of stay will undermine NHS Trusts' attempts at greater throughput. It is therefore important that the implications for hospital acquired infection control are carefully considered as part of all NHS Trusts bed management policies.

Conclusions and recommendations

3.37 Surveillance is the foundation for good infection control practice. We found examples of good practice in the way individual NHS Trusts have developed their own surveillance. We also welcome the development of the Nosocomial Infection

National Surveillance Scheme as key to improving patient care through identifying and reducing the extent of avoidable hospital acquired infection. Given that the majority of NHS Trusts consider that there is scope to reduce hospital acquired infection on average by 15 per cent (paragraph 3.2), and that this might produce gross savings for the NHS of as much as £150 million, there is significant scope to do more to reduce hospital acquired infection. We recommend that:

The Department should:

- emphasise the importance of surveillance and build on the success to date of the Nosocomial Infection National Surveillance Scheme, making improvements to it where possible while maintaining the emphasis on the achievement of its objectives to reduce infection rates by disseminating information on best practice;

- encourage participation in the Nosocomial Infection National Surveillance Scheme so that it becomes a comprehensive NHS scheme, facilitating the production of comparable data on infection rates;

- consider the need for post discharge surveillance to be carried out, either as part of a NHS Trust's own surveillance, or as a future module of the Nosocomial Infection National Surveillance Scheme;

- work with the Public Health Laboratory Service to evaluate and develop the Nosocomial Infection National Surveillance Scheme and consider other similar schemes, for example the USA National Nosocomial Infection Surveillance Scheme, to identify any lessons that might be applicable; and

- develop evidence based guidance on the cost effectiveness of intervention measures to reduce hospital acquired infection, and if necessary commission further research. The Department then needs to disseminate the results to NHS Trusts to ensure that they have the evidence-based information needed to determine the best approach to reduce the extent of hospital acquired infections.

NHS Trusts should:

- consider the level of resources required to undertake surveillance effectively and evaluate the benefits of providing such resources;

- ensure that there are appropriate mechanisms for feedback of surveillance data to clinicians, the Hospital Infection Control Committee etc and require evidence that these results are being acted on;

- when participating in the Nosocomial Infection National Surveillance Scheme, ensure that reasons for markedly worse than average performance are identified and acted upon;

- consider some form of post-discharge surveillance, either as part of the Nosocomial Infection National Surveillance Scheme or as part of the Trust's own surveillance;

- ensure that infection control considerations are an integral part of bed management policies; and

- assess their local situation to evaluate infection risks and implement those intervention measures which they believe would have the largest impact in reducing hospital acquired infection.

Part 4: The effectiveness of infection control practices and procedures

4.1 This part of the report examines how infection control teams discharge their infection control responsibilities, the extent to which current practices and procedures employed by infection control teams comply with Departmental guidelines and their effectiveness in preventing, detecting and controlling hospital acquired infections.

4.2 In addition to surveillance, the Department's guidance[9] and the Standards in Hospital Infection Control[14] identify the following as the other main prevention, detection and control measures:

(i) education and training of NHS Trust staff to inform them of procedures for infection control (paragraphs 4.4-4.8);

(ii) the development, dissemination and application of infection control policies and procedures (paragraphs 4.9-4.19);

(iii) monitoring and audit of hospital hygiene to ensure that the hospital environment is maintained in a way that minimises the potential for infectious agents to develop and spread (paragraphs 4.20-4.22);

(iv) clinical audit of infection control measures (paragraphs 4.23-4.28);

(v) contributing to decisions on purchase of equipment, plans for alterations and additions to buildings, and letting of catering and laundry service contracts (paragraphs 4.29-4.30); and

(vi) documented arrangements for dealing with infections including outbreak control, targeted screening and isolation of patients (paragraphs 4.31-4.41).

4.3 In response to our census, infection control teams felt they should be spending more time on proactive activities such as education and training and audit activities as this would have a greater impact on the prevention and control of hospital acquired infection. However, many infection control teams considered that most of their time was reactive, spent dealing with patients who either entered hospital with an infection or have acquired one since admission.

(i) Education and training

Not all clinical and other hospital staff receive training in infection control from the infection control team

4.4 The majority of infection control teams told us that education and training can be a powerful means of reducing infection rates. Case Study 7 shows how one NHS Trust has concentrated its efforts on this. Departmental guidance states that the infection control teams should provide an education programme for all hospital employees and students, but compliance varies widely. We found important gaps in the provision of induction education and training and in the extent to which key health care staff receive annual updates on infection control. For example:

■ 90 per cent of infection control teams provide induction training to nurses and health care assistants, but 10 per cent of NHS Trusts do not. Annual update training for nurses is provided in only 63 per cent of NHS Trusts, and for health care assistants in 53 per cent of NHS Trusts. Given that the main role of these staff is to deliver day to day hands on patient care, the absence of any induction training in 10 per cent of NHS Trusts together with the absence of regular updates causes some risk;

■ while 83 per cent of infection control teams provide induction training for junior doctors, only 16 per cent of infection control teams provide senior doctors with any induction training on infection control. Only 12 per cent of senior doctors are provided with annual updates. This is potentially serious as senior doctors are likely to be performing surgery and other invasive techniques, in which good infection control practice can have significant benefits;

■ other significant omissions in induction training provided by infection control teams for staff who have direct dealings with patients and who should be educated in good infection control practices from the outset include: cleaners (32 per cent of NHS Trusts do not provide induction training), food handling staff (41 per cent of NHS Trusts), nursing students (30 per cent of NHS Trusts) and medical students (45 per cent of NHS Trusts); and

■ thirty six infection control teams believed that staff education and training had led to reductions in hospital acquired infection. Five linked reductions to handwashing campaigns and three believed that ward audits had led to a reduction.

Case Study 7

Intensive education programme increased compliance with good infection control practices - North Manchester Healthcare NHS Trust

A detailed education and training programme with follow up audit of compliance has resulted in a notable reduction in infection. The Infection Control Team's Education Programme comprises:

■ Induction for new Trust employees. Direct and indirect carers are given an infection control lecture as part of their induction programme. This is evaluated in terms of relevance and knowledge gained by inductees and fed back to the Infection Control Team by the course organiser.

■ Yearly infection control updates on current issues and basic infection control training are given to domestic staff and porters. A link trainer has been named and is responsible for continuous basic infection control input to domestics. Performance is evaluated through environmental audit involving the Infection Control Team and continual observation audits.

■ Medical students and nursing staff shadow the Infection Control Team as part of their educational programmes. The role of the Infection Control Team is discussed. The educational value is evaluated and fed back to the Infection Control Team by course leaders.

■ There is a large input of formal teaching from the Infection Control Team on National Vocational Programmes (NVQ) levels I and II. This is evaluated by formal audits, observational audit in clinical areas and feedback to the NVQ course leader.

■ A rolling programme of education to NHS Trust nursing staff is carried out in all clinical areas on a 12 month basis. This includes current issues in infection control and evidence based practice. It is evaluated by observational audit and formal audit, for example isolation audit.

■ There is a programme of formal teaching provided by the Infection Control Team to Manchester University students undertaking: Communicable Disease MSc; ENB 329; ENB Medical Module; ENB 210; Project 2000 nursing course, BSc in nursing; MSc in Microbiology; and Diploma in Bacteriology. Formal teaching is also provided to link nurses in the community and Manchester Social Services care workers. The input is evaluated by course organisers and fed back to the team.

Note: Information provided by the Infection Control Team at North Manchester Healthcare NHS Trust and validated through NAO audit visit and review of relevant documents.

4.5 Overall, we consider that provision of effective education and training is a key measure in the prevention of hospital acquired infection but that the current provision falls below the basic requirement indicated in the Departmental guidance, namely that all staff should be provided with education in infection control procedures. We recognised that activity to prevent, control and treat infection in hospital takes place at many different levels as part of the day to day work of doctors, nurses and other professional health care staff. Also that these staff take a personal and professional responsibility for routinely adopting good infection control practice. Indeed many of these staff will have received some infection control training as part of their basic qualification. However, given the importance of education and training in relation to infection control, we would reiterate the Department's 1995 guidance[9] that all infection control teams need to ensure that they establish an education programme for all employees and students. As a first priority, they should target those staff who have direct contact with patients.

4.6 A few infection control teams suggested that training in infection control should be given the same mandatory status as Health and Safety training. While this proposition was not pursued further during this study, there may be some merit in the NHS Executive exploring this possibility further to obtain wider views on the advantages and disadvantages of such action.

Only forty nine per cent of the NHS Trusts had audited the effectiveness of their training

4.7 It is important that education and training is delivered effectively. But audits to evaluate the effectiveness of education and training on infection control had been carried out in only 49 per cent of NHS Trusts. Most of these were within the last three years. The results of these audits varied. In twenty NHS Trusts the results were satisfactory noting steady, general levels of improvement in infection control practice following training courses, but in others the problems identified included:

■ unsatisfactory levels of compliance, particularly in relation to hygiene standards;

■ insufficient education programmes to provide learning re-enforcement;

■ lack of adherence to handwashing procedures; and

■ poor practice in sharps disposal and improper assembly/positioning of sharps boxes.

To improve access to up to date information and advice on infection control, some NHS Trusts have developed infection control Assisted Learning Packages

4.8 Infection control teams' ability to deliver training is limited by the amount of time they have available to run the training course and the constraint of other staff finding the time to attend training sessions. The Infection Control Team at Kings College Hospital, Case Study 8, have addressed this problem by developing their own Interactive Computer Assisted Learning Training Package. This package has been adopted by a number of other NHS Trusts. There are also some commercial infection control CD ROM packages available on the market which, at the time of the National Audit Office census, were being tested by a number of NHS Trusts. These approaches offer a cost-effective way of addressing the weaknesses in training and education.

Case study 8

Development of infection control Computer Assisted Learning Software at King's College Hospital

The academic group and the infection control team at King's College Hospital developed and implemented a computerised multimedia 'Introduction to Infection Control' training module. It allowed staff to recognise how, when and why infection control problems may occur; identify areas where the risk of infection for both patients and staff can be reduced; and gain a basic understanding of some micro-organisms of particular concern within the hospital.

No formal training was given on the use of the software. Posters explaining how to start and use the programme were sent to ward managers, and technical support was available in the computer room. The effectiveness of the training module was assessed using a pre and post use questionnaire, and by comparison with medical students who attended a lecture covering the same content as the training module. A file that logs the number of users was monitored monthly for 18 months and twice daily for a four week period.

Staff and students were very positive about the ease of use, navigation and other user interface design issues of the program. Nursing Grades A to D, who spent more than half an hour going through the module, indicated that their knowledge of the topic had increased significantly, though all staff wanted more questions and answers built into the module to test their learning.

continued...

Case study 8 continued

The pattern of usage was highest on night duty and at week-ends. The module was accessed 3,101 times on the hospital network in 18 months with usage settling to between 100 and 150 times per month. The sustained number of users over the 18 month trial period indicated that ward staff were using and learning from the program regularly. Staff were also printing out the certificate, available at the end of the test quiz, and displaying them in the wards. This generated peer pressure and discussion and debate and increased awareness of infection control. The NHS Trust's Infection Control Manual has since been added to the package allowing ready access to this information throughout the hospital.

The cost of the Infection Control Training and Policies package (IC-TAP) is similar to the previously incurred cost of updating and redistributing revised copies of the Infection Control Manual.

(ii) Policies and procedures to address hospital acquired infection

Not all NHS Trusts had comprehensive written policies and procedures for the prevention of infection

4.9 A second infection control activity which infection control teams undertake to help prevent and control hospital acquired infection is the production and dissemination of up to date infection control policies and procedures. The recently published Departmental guidance on controls assurances[21] reaffirms the need for every hospital to have written policies, procedures and guidelines for the prevention and control of infection, and that they are reviewed regularly.

4.10 Almost all NHS Trusts had policies and procedures in place for dealing with MRSA, patient isolation, handling of sharps and clinical waste management. However we found that:

- eight per cent of NHS Trusts did not have a written policy on handwashing, regarded by many as a highly effective way to prevent hospital acquired infection;

- ten per cent of NHS Trusts did not have a written antibiotic policy, which we consider makes them vulnerable given the increase in antibiotic resistance. In some cases the antibiotic policies have been revised recently to reflect evidence from analysing trend data (Case Study 9); and

- over a quarter of NHS Trusts did not have written policies on the use of urinary catheters or intravascular devices which is a significant omission given that numerous studies and articles have shown these to be high risk procedures in relation to hospital acquired infection.

Case Study 9

Revision to antibiotic policy based on statistical analysis of cases of *Clostridium difficile* compared with the use of injectable cephalosporins between April 1993 and March 1999 at the Whittington NHS Trust

In 1994, the Infection Control Doctor at the Whittington Hospital identified *Clostridium difficile* as a major cause of morbidity particularly amongst the elderly. The number of cases were again higher than expected in the first half of 1997. Statistical evidence of improvement was seen in April 1998. Some of the factors seen as bringing about these improvements were staff education and awareness, together with improved cleaning but the main reason for the increase in cases was demonstrably linked to the rise in the use of the antibiotic cephalosporin and the improvement was due to a change in antibiotic use.

There is scope to streamline the production and update of NHS Trust's Infection Control Manuals

4.11 Most infection control teams have combined their policies and procedures in an Infection Control Manual. This enables the principles of good infection control practice to be combined in one document and eases access. We found that 95 per cent of NHS Trust infection control teams had developed their own infection control manual and a further 3 per cent were preparing theirs at the time of our census. Over half of these manuals had been updated in the last six months and a further 21 per cent within the last 12 months. However, in 8 per cent of NHS Trusts, the manual had not been updated in the previous four years, which means that they are seriously out of date particularly with regard to the Departmental guidance issued in 1995 and more recent developments.

4.12 Many infection control teams commented on the large amount of time consumed in updating their manual and the difficulties of ensuring that, once updated, it was readily accessible to and accessed by staff. One Infection Control Doctor commented that it had taken three years to develop a manual for his NHS Trust. Because each infection control team develops its own infection control manual, we found considerable evidence of "re-inventing the wheel". While we understand the need to have policies and procedures tailored to local needs, there are many policies and procedures that could be applied to all hospitals.

4.13 We consider there is merit in the approach taken by the Scottish Office, which issued a single infection control manual in 1998[28], providing "guidance on core standards for the control of infection in hospital, health care premises and the community interface". It is issued and will be amended centrally. All Health Boards and hospitals in Scotland are expected to conform to it.

Infection Control Manuals are not used as widely as they should be

4.14 In our visits to NHS Trusts, we found that infection control manuals are not easily accessible. This means that a potential source of information and education, which took a lot of effort to develop, is not being fully utilised. A number of factors reduce the use of manuals, such as insufficient number of copies, staff not knowing where copies are kept, or staff finding that bulky volumes are off-putting.

4.15 Information technology can help provide a solution. Where the manual has been converted into electronic format, it improves both access and the speed and reliability of accessing up to date relevant information. It can also be used as a monitoring tool to evaluate the extent to which guidance is being accessed. For example in Scunthorpe and Goole NHS Trust the manual has been put onto the hospital intranet, nursing and ward aides are given around 45 minutes training and then allowed to access it as and when needed. An analysis of use shows that the web site has been accessed more than 4,000 times in the last 12 months. In addition, the costs involved in updating manuals held electronically are relatively small and result in efficiency gains as it can be done at source, in comparison to updating manuals which requires time consuming production of large numbers of amendments, and there is no guarantee that they are then incorporated into the manual.

Infection control doctor and infection control nurse providing advice on use of infection control web site to paediatric nurse

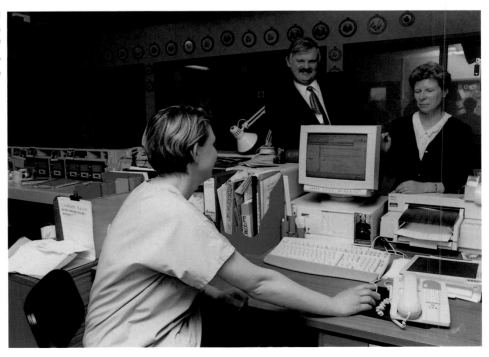

Proper handwashing is an effective preventative hygiene measure, but one that is not always observed

4.16 Published articles suggest that effective hand hygiene is possibly the most important factor in preventing hospital acquired infection but that compliance is poor[29][30][31]. Figures 22a and 22b illustrate how handwashing techniques can be improved. A number of studies have generated data that confirm that doctors who decontaminate their hands between seeing patients reduce hospital infection rates. Yet many observational studies, mainly conducted in intensive care units, show low rates of hand washing especially among doctors. Insufficient washbasins, supplies of liquid soap and paper towels, are some of the reasons that have been given for this.

Results of ineffective handwashing

Figure 22a

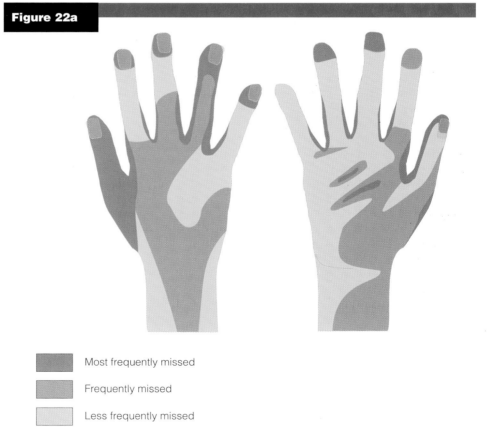

Most frequently missed

Frequently missed

Less frequently missed

Source: Nursing Times

Ineffective handwashing techniques result in some areas of the hands consistently being missed, facilitating cross infection by transient bacteria.

Figure 22b — Practical procedures for handwashing

Effective handwashing procedures can remove all transient bacteria. The adoption of this simple but effective technique has been demonstrated to significantly reduce rates of hospital acquired infection.

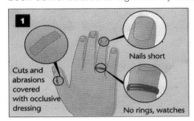

Some general points need emphasising: Keep nails short; avoid wearing rings and watches; cover cuts and abrasions with occlusive waterproof dressings to reduce the risk of bloodborne infection such as hepatitis B, C and HIV.

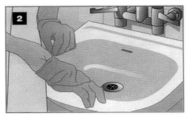

Hands should be decontaminated even if gloves have been worn - they may be punctured or leak. Even if the gloves are intact, hands can become contaminated as the gloves are removed. A sink with elbow or foot-operated taps should be used if at all possible.

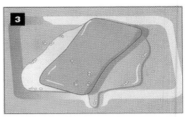

Dispensers for soaps and skin disinfectants should be designed to prevent contamination of the contents when they are handled. Bars of soap become contaminated easily and contribute to the risks of cross-infection.

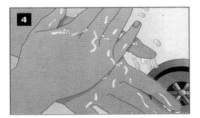

Effective decontamination technique starts with dispensing soap or skin disinfectant onto the moistened hands. Rub the palms together vigorously to aid the removal of dead cells and bacteria.

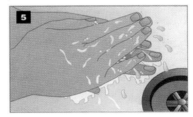

Ensure hand surfaces receive contact. It helps to have a set routine - always decontaminate the dorsal surface after the palms.

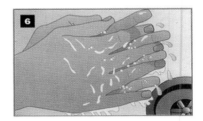

Remember to decontaminate the interdigital spaces as they are often heavily contaminated.

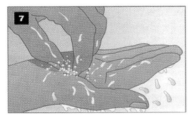

Decontaminate the fingertips of each hand in turn to create friction against the palm of the opposing hand.

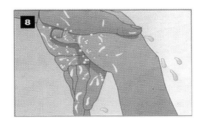

Clasp the hands together, ensuring that thumbs and wrists receive contact with each other.

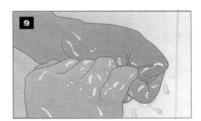

Avoid splashing during the hand decontamination routine so as to avoid contaminating clothing and the surrounding environment.

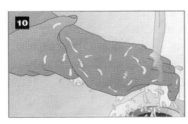

Rinse all hand surfaces thoroughly: residual soap or antiseptic can make the skin sore and dry. After thorough rinsing turn the tap off by the elbows or feet. Take care not to recontaminate the hands by touching the tap.

Source: Nursing Times

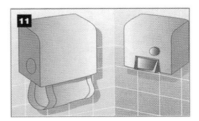

As wet surfaces transfer micro-organisms more effectively than dry ones, always dry the hands thoroughly with a paper towel. Communal towels promote cross-infection, while driers circulate air loaded with bacteria.

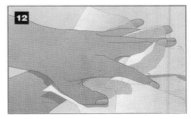

Friction caused by the hands on the paper towel helps to remove remaining bacteria. In the community, it may be necessary to carry paper towels to homes where hand decontamination facilities are inadequate.

4.17 However, access to adequate handwashing facilities does not guarantee compliance. Most of the NHS Trusts in our census had run handwashing campaigns and stressed the need for the commitment of senior staff in promoting better hand hygiene and monitoring (Case Study10). A significant number of NHS Trusts also reported that while there was usually an immediate improvement, the impact of their campaign reduced within a short period of time. Some infection control doctors consider that handwashing campaigns need to be repeated every six months or so.

Case Study 10

Handwashing campaign run by the Leeds Teaching Hospital NHS Trust in 1998

Problem

For several years the large and busy neo-natal unit has had a problem with an endemic MSSA (Methicillin Sensitive *Staphylococcus Aureus*). The Infection Control Team made rigorous attempts at control and eradication, including screening staff and babies several times, introducing additional infection control measures, education campaigns, environment and practice audits, and the introduction of cosmetically acceptable soap and an alcohol gel to encourage hand hygiene. These all had some measures of success. However periodic clusters of infection/colonisation continued to appear, usually at busy times of the year.

Solution

The Hospital decided to concentrate mainly on the likely method of spread, ie hands. The unit's senior consultant and senior nursing staff were keen to make hand hygiene a top priority and act as champions and role models, and ensure that all staff were empowered to point out lapses in any other staff member's hand hygiene. The Infection Control Team did random anonymised hand impressions on plates, the results of which were fed back to the ward in written and photographic form. The team also produced posters that said "**If I haven't washed my hands, please tell me; if you haven't washed yours I'll tell you**".

Hand impressions on agar plates showing result of effective handwashing (left plate) compared with ineffective handwashing (right plate)

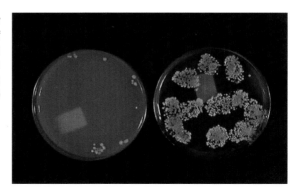

continued...

Case Study 10 continued

Outcome   Over the first six weeks of the campaign there were no isolations of the endemic organism, despite activity on the unit remaining high. The Infection Control Team feels that this demonstrates the importance of hand hygiene in preventing the spread of infection. The commitment of the most senior staff in promoting good hand hygiene was recognised. It was also vital to create an atmosphere in which staff can remind everyone, no matter how senior, to follow and continue following best practice.

4.18   In recognition of the problems with handwashing, in March 1999, a Handwashing Liaison Group (comprising: the Hospital Infection Society, Association of Medical Microbiologists, Department of Health, Infection Control Nurses Association, Royal Colleges of Nursing and Public Health Laboratory Service) issued an Action Plan on handwashing[32]. The Department of Health sent this document to all NHS chief executives, public health directors and microbiologists in England.

4.19   The Liaison Group[32] recommends policies that endorse the development of good role models, which are supported by chief executives, and details a set of action points for NHS Trusts. Given the results of our census and the strong views expressed to us about the importance of handwashing, and the problems of compliance, we strongly endorse the initiative and the recommendations of the Liaison Group.

(iii) Monitoring hospital hygiene

There is scope to increase the infection control team's role in monitoring hospital hygiene

4.20   Good hygiene practices are a further set of preventative measures specified in the Department's 1995 guidance[9]. This guidance requires infection control teams to collaborate with other relevant staff in monitoring the implementation and effectiveness of the hospital's routine procedures on: cleaning, housekeeping, disinfection or sterilisation of instruments and equipment, production of sterile supplies, safe collection and disposal of clinical waste, kitchen hygiene, control of legionellae, control of insects and vermin etc. The aim of this monitoring is to help prevent hospital acquired infection.

4.21 Evidence to the House of Lords Select Committee inquiry on Antibiotic Resistance[24] strongly supported the view that standards in hospital hygiene are slipping. Poor hygiene was implicated in some outbreaks of hospital infection and the Infection Control Nurses Association were especially concerned about cleaning of hospital wards. A recent Infection Control Nurse Association survey identified serious shortcomings in hospital hygiene.[33]

4.22 Our census shows that eighty five per cent of infection control teams have carried out environmental audits of hospital hygiene. But while 89 per cent of audits had covered clinical waste management and 88 per cent cleaning, fewer (81 per cent) covered the key area of handwashing, and only two thirds covered domestic services. While we feel that audit work is not presently meeting guidelines in full, infection control teams pointed to a number of changes that have taken place in response to their audit reports (Figure 23). The overall view of infection control teams was that an audit cycle involving: identifying the problem; relevant education and training; action plan; and re-audit led to visible improvements in preventing infection.

Infection control nurses providing advice to staff on cleaning and need for effective sterilisation of equipment

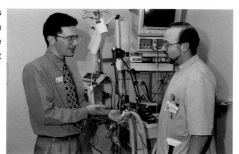
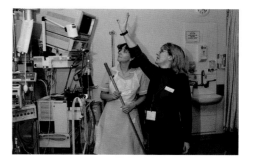

Results of environmental audits by infection control teams

Figure 23	
Details of change in activity response to environmental audit reports	**Number of Infection Control Teams introducing change**
Improved practices/approach to ward cleaning	47
Improved clinical waste disposal procedures and segregation of clinical and other waste	34
Improved/upgraded handwashing facilities and policies including introduction of liquid soap and handwashing awareness campaigns	30
Improved sharps management including new design and placement of sharps bins	25
Increased emphasis on food hygiene, including education and training, also increase in kitchen inspections	25
Better monitoring of ward refridgerators including refridgerator thermometers	16
Repairs to broken taps/showers/surfaces and tiles	13
Improved mattress replacement policies	13

Source: National Audit Office Census

(iv) Clinical audit of infection control measures

Over two thirds of infection control teams input into the standard setting and audit of clinical and support services

4.23 The infection control team's position with regard to clinical audit is complex in that its responsibilities for infection control encompass the whole hospital. The team is therefore required to contribute, to some extent, to the standard setting and audit for a range of clinical and support services as well as setting it's own standards and auditing it's own activities.

4.24 Departmental guidance[9] states that the infection control team should collaborate with other staff in the production of detailed standards, policies and procedures and in the development of audit tools for these and should support the audit process. While only half of infection control teams specifically included audit in their annual infection control programme, many of the infection control teams in the census acknowledged that audit was an important part of the cycle to improve control of infection. The importance of audit has increased as a result of the Government's initiative on clinical governance[19].

4.25 Sixty five per cent of infection control teams told us that they had contributed to the audit process and 75 per cent of teams that they had contributed to the standard setting process. During 1997-98, the main focus of the infection control teams input to clinical audit was in relation to the arrangements for the control of MRSA, followed by surgical wound audit, safe handling of sharps and antibiotic prescribing. As a result of these audits, infection control teams identified a need for specific training to re-emphasise the importance of various infection control activities such as: sharps policy (41 NHS Trusts); antibiotic prescribing (26 NHS Trusts); isolation practice (20 NHS Trusts) and MRSA policies and procedures (12 NHS Trusts).

Less than a fifth of infection control teams actively evaluate their own performance

4.26 Departmental guidelines require infection control teams to set standards for assessing their own performance. These standards should cover the scope and quality of surveillance and the scope and frequency of infection control education provided. Other performance indicators are the management of infection outbreaks, speed of response to incidents and the provision of 24 hour care. However, only 19 per cent of infection control teams had carried out a clinical audit of their own activities and it is difficult to reach any general conclusions on effectiveness from these audits. Given the range of responsibilities of the infection control team, it is essential that there is some measure of the impact of their work in preventing, detecting and controlling infection to demonstrate their effectiveness to NHS Trust management.

In some NHS Trusts audit has influenced practice and led to reductions in infection and lower costs

4.27 A number of infection control teams supplied details of interventions that they believed had reduced rates of hospital acquired infection and which had achieved demonstrable cost savings. The main areas cited were in relation to *Methiculin Resistant Stophylococcus Aureus (MRSA)* and *Clostridium diffiicle*, particularly in the care of the elderly. Fifty one out of 110 NHS Trusts indicated that a change in antibiotic policy had helped control *Clostridium difficile* and a similar number identified active management of MRSA including revision in antibiotic prescribing, as preventing the problem (Case study 11). Fourteen infection control teams mentioned that they had achieved reductions in infection due to revised policies on central intravascular devices and urinary catheters.

Case Study 11

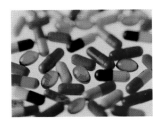

Changing antibiotic policy to reduce hospital acquired infection has led to demonstrable cost savings

(A) Change in antibiotic policy at Scunthorpe and Goole NHS Trust

Concerns over increasing levels of *Clostridium difficile* associated diarrhoea in elderly patients culminated in 20 new cases in one ward over three days. Following an outbreak control meeting the Infection Control Doctor developed a new antibiotic policy that recommended ceasing to use Cephlasphorins on the wards and recommended suitable alternatives for different infections. To support the proposed change in policy, the infection control team mounted an education awareness campaign. They targeted doctors through posters in wards, giving advice on what antibiotics to use and when. As a result of this campaign and change to the antibiotic policy there was a dramatic reduction in the incidence of *Clostridium difficile* infection with the number of new cases on the Care of the Elderly ward decreasing from 163 in 1996-97 to 20 in 1997-98. It was demonstrated that the extra cost of the new antibiotic policy, estimated at £12,192 per annum, was more than offset by reducing the numbers of *Clostridium difficile* infections, estimated as around £278,000 per annum (based on associated length of stay data). There were also perceived reductions in morbidity and possibly mortality though the full extent has not been measured.

(B) Change in antibiotic policy at Addensbrooke NHS Trust

A change in the antibiotic policy at Addenbrookes NHS Trust, for the treatment of elderly patients with *Clostridium difficile*, led to a 50 per cent reduction in the number of cases of infectious diarrhoea (53 fewer cases). While acknowledging that cost savings are difficult to quantify, attempts were made to calculate savings using data calculated for the hospital and published in 1996-97.[34] This study calculated that patients with *Clostridium difficile* diarrhoea stay on in hospital 20.5 days extra (39.5 days versus 19 days for controls). Using an estimated cost of a bed of £150-£200 per day and some additional costs for diagnostic tests, antibiotics, etc, this represented an additional cost of approximately £4,000 per case of *Clostridium difficile*. The 53 fewer cases therefore represented a potential saving of 1,087 bed days (53 x 20.5) or £212,000 [53 x £4,000]. While this may not represent actual cost savings there is evidence that it reduced mortality, morbidity and bed occupancy.[35]

(C) Change in approach at the Norfolk and Norwich NHS Trust reduced infection rates in vascular graft patients and also saved money

The Norfolk and Norwich NHS Trust's change in its measures aimed at the control of infection in vascular graft patients led to a reduction in infection rates from 30 per cent to 12 per cent over the course of 15 months. Those due to MRSA fell from 13 per cent to 5 per cent and non MRSA from 17 per cent to 7 per cent, per annum. The costs of the change included £1,000 for change in antibiotic prophylaxis, £500 for use of pre-op wash, and £6,000 for MRSA screening. This cost increase of £7,500, compared with the estimated reduced length of stay costs of £195,000 per annum.

4.28 Some NHS Trusts provided information on prevention activities that they had stopped, because they had found that they were not effective, Case Study 12 and Figure 24.

Case Study 12

Change in type of handwash and gloves at the Homerton Hospital led to cash saving

The Infection Control Team proposed changing the type of handwash gel in day to day use in clinical areas throughout the hospital. They considered that one product appeared to be more expensive than products currently in use, but larger quantities of the latter were needed to achieve effective handwashing. The total cost of changing the handwash gel and changing the type of gloves used, resulted in a projected saving of £35,000 per annum.

Examples of activities NHS Trusts found had no effect on controlling infection

Figure 24

■ Routine use of disinfectants for ward cleaning (24 NHS Trusts) - one NHS Trust, Stoke Mandeville, estimated that stopping the use of disinfectants saved £20,000 in one year,

■ Use of over-shoes in theatres (6 NHS Trusts);

■ Masks and hats in outer theatre or for wound dressing (6 NHS Trusts);

■ Use of gowns by visitors to theatre (5 NHS Trusts);

■ Normal three dose antibiotic prophylaxis was no more effective than single dose (4 NHS Trusts);

■ Turning operating theatre ventilation off at night was quoted by two NHS Trusts as saving £8,900 and £16,000-£20,000 per annum respectively; and

Source: National Audit Office Census

■ Reducing the use of sterile gloves in non-invasive procedures was mentioned by 3 NHS Trusts as leading to estimated savings of £10,000, £8,000 and £50,000 respectively.

(v) Wider involvement of infection control teams

More involvement of infection control teams in the wider support activities of the NHS Trust could aid prevention of infection

4.29 The Department's 1995 guidance[9] require infection control teams to be involved in discussions about:

■ the purchase of equipment;

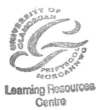

■ plans for alterations and additions to the building; and

■ the letting of catering and laundry service contracts to ensure that infection control is given due consideration.

All of these activities have implications for preventing and controlling infection in hospitals. The lack of involvement in activities within a hospital can have serious implications for infection control. Figure 25 details the extent of involvement by infection control teams in the wider activities of the NHS Trusts. It shows that there is much more scope to involve infection control teams across all of the activities specified in the Departmental guidance.

4.30 The new Controls Assurance Standards for Infection Control[21] emphasises the importance of obtaining infection control advice from the infection control team, particularly in relation to engineering and building services, purchase of medical devices and equipment and all stages of contracting for catering, cleaning, laundry and clinical waste services. Compliance with these standards should help address the shortcomings identified in Figure 25.

Extent of consultation/involvement of the infection control team in NHS Trust support activities

Figure 25

The involvement of infection control teams in support activities that impact on infection control is varied. Most Infection control teams are consulted in purchasing equipment or making alterations to buildings and few are never consulted. While between a quarter and a third of NHS Trusts always consult their infection control team when reviewing the contracts for catering, laundry or domestic services, a similar number never involve them.

Non-medical activity	Always	Most times	Sometimes	Never	Not stated
Purchase of new equipment	2%	21%	71%	6%	1%
Building Plans	8%	40%	48%	3%	1%
Catering Services	23%	16%	22%	35%	4%
Laundry Services	35%	18%	24%	23%	0%
Domestic and Cleaning Services	31%	20%	25%	25%	1%

Source: National Audit Office Census

(vi) Documented arrangements for dealing with infections, including outbreak control, targeted screening and isolation of patients

NHS Trusts are required to have adequately documented arrangements for controlling outbreaks

4.31 The final component of infection prevention, detection and control involves the need for documented protocols for managing outbreaks. The key points of a good outbreak control plan are:

- the infection control team, in liaison with the Consultant in Communicable Disease Control, is responsible for drawing up detailed plans, appropriate to the local situation, for the management of incidents and outbreaks in the hospital;

- these plans should be discussed and endorsed by the Hospital Infection Control Committee and should include the criteria and method for convening an Outbreak Control Group which, when necessary, will be expanded into a Major Outbreak Control Group;

- assignments of lead responsibility to the Infection Control Doctor or Consultant in Communicable Disease Control;

- local authority Environmental Health Officers must also be informed promptly of any infectious incidents where food or water is involved; and

- at the end of any outbreak a short report must be prepared by the infection control team and circulated to all members of the Outbreak Control Group, if convened, and to the Consultant in Communicable Disease Control and Hospital Infection Control Committee.

4.32 The rapid detection of outbreaks is one of the objectives of surveillance. Once a possible outbreak has been recognised the Infection Control Doctor is the person primarily responsible for action within the hospital.

4.33 All infection control teams confirmed that they had documented arrangements for dealing with outbreaks and incidents of hospital acquired infection. However in 3 per cent of NHS Trusts they had not been discussed with the Hospital Infection Control Committee and in 5 per cent they had not been endorsed by this Committee. It is important that such endorsements be obtained in all cases so that all concerned are content with the arrangements put in place.

4.34 Written reports on each outbreak appear to have been prepared in only 76 per cent of NHS Trusts, and only 64 per cent of NHS Trusts normally complied with Departmental guidance and sent them to the Consultant in Communicable Disease Control, and 79% to the Hospital Infection Control Committee. The failure to follow Departmental guidance means that some valuable lessons may not be learned, putting patients at greater risk. The reasons for this departure from the guidance were not clear from our census.

More evidence on the cost effectiveness of screening is needed

4.35 Screening involves taking swabs from symptomatic patients and staff which are then subjected to microbiological testing to determine whether they are colonised or infected by specific micro-organisms. While patients can be screened for any infection, the main focus of regular screening by NHS Trusts was for MRSA. We found that some infection control teams saw screening patients as an infection control measure that had been successful in reducing MRSA infection rates in their NHS Trust and there has been a notable rise in screening susceptible patients for MRSA. For example, Kings College Hospital have set up a process dedicated to screening for MRSA, with some 15,000 tests carried out each year costing about £120,000 per annum. They told us that they consider this to be a cost effective measure in reducing infection rates. Other NHS Trusts have used screening in a cost effective way in high risk situations (see Case Study 13).

Agar plate showing
Staphylococcus
aureus

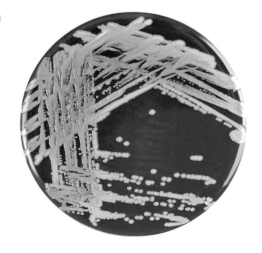

Case Study 13	**Management of MRSA in Hip Prosthesis patients at Frimley Park Hospital**

Problem   In 1994 the NHS Trust had an outbreak of MRSA which led to six hip transplant patients acquiring a deep wound infection. All of these patients required replacement hips and spent several years requiring follow up care. Some of these patients are still returning to the hospital for treatment five years later. The estimated costs of managing these patients (excluding repeat surgery and return visits) was £20,000.

Solution   The NHS Trust agreed that the Infection Control Team should adopt a policy of actively screening all hip prosthesis patients. If the patient is found to be MRSA positive, they are given an antibiotic prophylaxis which is known to combat the particular strain of infection (ie teicoplanin, which is very expensive but known to work on MRSA). In addition the patient is placed in an isolation ward if possible. If an isolation room is not available the patient will be cohort nursed with other patients who are MRSA positive.

Outcome   As a result of the Infection Control Team adopting a combination of detection and control measures, namely active screening, rapid feedback of results, rapid treatment and isolation, the NHS Trust orthopaedic unit has seen a significant reduction in the number of infections in the last 3 years.

4.36   However, screening patients is expensive and a number of infection control teams questioned whether it was always of value. Indeed, 22 infection control teams stated that actively screening patients, other than in high risk situations, had no impact on their infection rates. While there is guidance on screening in high risk situations, there is no guidance about screening in general. A number of NHS Trusts identified the need for evidence based research to inform their screening policies, to determine when it is likely to be cost effective.

4.37   There is also little evidence about the benefits of screening staff for MRSA. Seventy two NHS Trusts specifically highlighted blanket screening of staff for MRSA as having no impact on their NHS Trust's hospital acquired infection rates. They noted that it caused unnecessary distress for staff, and significant problems for occupational health staff who had to manage staff found to be positive. There was a general view that staff screening, other than in high dependency units, should be discontinued.

Many infection control teams consider that facilities for isolation of infected patients are unsatisfactory, but some NHS Trusts have recently been successful in increasing isolation facilities

4.38 The House of Lords Select Committee report[10] states that "Isolation of patients is an expensive but effective form of infection control". Patients may be nursed in isolation if they have a disease or condition that has the potential to spread or because they are highly susceptible to acquiring an infection as a result of their underlying condition or therapy. Isolation of patients may be required on admission of a patient with a particular infection in order to prevent the spread to in-patients, and for those patients who develop an infection during their hospital stay. There are two main categories of isolation. The first, protective isolation, aims to shield the immuno-compromised patient from pathogens or micro-organisms that may be acquired from health workers, family and friends, the environment or other patients. The second, source isolation, aims to prevent the transfer of pathogens or resistant organisms from infected or colonised patients to other patients and staff.

Infection control team members providing advice on injection control procedure to nursing staff in isolation facility

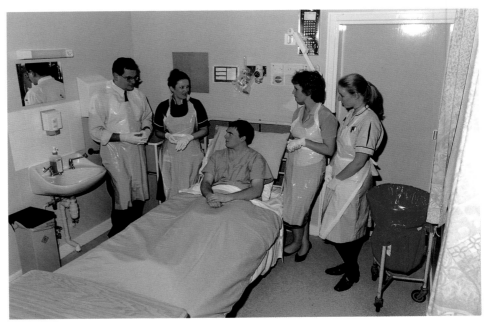

4.39 Isolation facilities in some NHS Trusts have been significantly reduced over the last five to six years[11], and some infection control teams believe this has created a serious problem, especially in their efforts to deal with MRSA, which is now endemic in many hospitals. We found that nearly a quarter of NHS Trusts have seen a decrease in the number of isolation side-rooms between April 1997 and March 1998, due in part to ward and bed closures, and alternative uses of the side-rooms, including use as office space. While 13 per cent of infection control teams were very satisfied and 41 per cent were fairly satisfied with their isolation facilities, over 40 per cent of infection control teams were either not very satisfied or not satisfied at all with their isolation facilities. There appears to have been little evaluation of the cost-effectiveness of closing isolation facilities.

4.40   Between April 1997 and March 1998 twenty four per cent of NHS Trusts have increased their isolation facilities. In particular, two per cent have increased the number of isolation wards, 7 per cent the number of side rooms and 11 per cent the number of negative pressure rooms. In addition, a number of NHS Trusts have prepared a business case arguing the case for a dedicated isolation ward (Case Study 14).

Case Study 14

Development of an isolation unit for Rotherham General Hospital NHS Trust

The NHS Trust had a limited number of isolation side-rooms which was causing problems, for example, beds being blocked in 6 bedded bays. Also, the majority of existing side-rooms lacked the en-suite facilities necessary to prevent the spread of infection.

The Infection Control Team with the support of the Bed manager prepared a business case, which:

■ demonstrated, using the widely quoted incidence and prevalence rates from published studies, the extent and impact of hospital acquired infection and pointed to the fact that, isolation facilities were inadequate to meet the demand in the NHS Trust, particularly as the NHS Trust was experiencing significant increases in MRSA, *Clostridium difficle* and Tuberculosis;

■ provided detailed evidence of problems caused by cross infection;

■ identified the advantages of a dedicated isolation unit, such as improved patient care, release of side rooms, lower risk of transmission within families visiting patients; reducing the risk of cancelled elective admissions, avoiding ward closures, and shorter length of stay, with greater eradication success;

■ stated how the unit would be managed;

■ presented appraisal of options of where the unit could be located, and a plan of the ward; and

■ estimated the cost of the unit as approximately £400,000.

Although widespread support for such a ward, the hospital is still in the process of identifying the most appropriate/relevant ward to pursue the plan. Following this, the business plan will be presented to the Hospital Management Board, under leadership of the Chief Executive, for approval.

The need for isolation facilities has not been fully assessed

4.41 The Department's 1995 guidance[9] states that "all general hospitals need to have isolation facilities available either in suitable side rooms on general wards or in separate isolation wards or both. Health and Safety at Work legislation requires hospital management to ensure that formal risk assessments are carried out and that arrangements are in place to minimise the risk of transmission of infection to patients and staff. The nature and extent of isolation facilities available needs to be considered as part of this assessment." We found that a third of NHS Trusts had carried out a formal risk assessment of the hospital environment to ensure that arrangements are in place to minimise the risk of transmission of infection to patients. A similar number of NHS Trusts had carried out an assessment of the risk of transmission to staff.

Conclusions and recommendations

4.42 Overall we found infection control teams to be a professional and dedicated group of NHS staff whose role and responsibilities have increased significantly over the last five years or so. We also found many examples of good practice in preventing and controlling hospital acquired infection. However, there is scope for further improvement particularly in relation to education and training and in the audit of compliance with infection control guidelines. We consider that:

The Department should

- consider the benefits of producing an Infection Control Manual as is the case in Scotland, with the possibility for local "add ons";

- consider the need for a revision of the 1995 guidance on Infection Control; and

- consider the available evidence on the cost effectiveness of screening patients and staff and on isolation of patients and develop standards and guidelines where appropriate.

Glycepeptide resistant enterococci	Enterococci bacteria that are resistant to glycepeptides. Such as Vancomycin and/or Teicoplanin.
Health care assistant	Support staff who are trained, or undertaking training in job related competencies through NVQs and other local training arrangements.
Hepatitis	Inflammation of the liver.
Hospital acquired infection	An infection that was neither present nor incubating at the time of a patient's admission to hospital (the definition used for this study is an infection that normally manifests itself more than three nights after the patient's admission to hospital).
Hospital Infection Control Committee	The main forum for routine consultation between the infection control team and the rest of the NHS Trust. It is required to approve and lend support to the infection control teams programme.
Hospital hygiene	The hospitals routine procedures on cleaning, housekeeping, disinfection, sterilisation of instruments, equipment, production of sterile supplies, safe collection and disposal of clinical waste, kitchen hygiene, control of insects, vermin, etc.
Inflammation	The response of tissues to damage caused by physical, chemical or biological agents
Immune	Being highly resistant to a disease due to the formation of antibodies, the development of immunological competent cells, or both as the result of another mechanism.
Immuno-compromised	A person who has impaired immunity due to disease (eg cancer) or treatment (eg radiotherapy).
Immuno-suppression	Prevent or impair the immune response by radiotherapy or drug therapy for example cancer treatment.
Incidence	The number of new events/episodes of a disease that occur in a population in a given time period.
Infection	Invasion and multiplication of harmful micro-organisms in body tissues.
Infection control doctor(s)	Normally a consultant medical microbiologist, with knowledge of aspects of infection control, which should include epidemiology. The infection control doctor normally provides leadership to the infection control team and is responsible to the NHS Trust chief executive for its work.

Infection control nurse(s)	Normally a registered general nurse with knowledge of all aspects of infection control.
Infection control team	A team within an NHS Trust which has prime responsibility for, and reports to the chief executive on, all aspects of surveillance prevention and control of infection. The members of the team are an infection control doctor and infection control nurse(s).
Infectious	Caused by or capable of being communicated by infection.
Intravascular (device)	Catheter/cannula inserted into a vein or artery.
Isolation precautions	Additional precautions to be taken with some patients/clients/residents, normally removing them and placing them away from normal contact with other people.
IT	Information technology such as computers.
Legionella	The bacterium that causes a pneumonia like disease in humans, eg legionnaires disease.
Legionnaires Disease	Form of bacterial pneumonia first identified after an outbreak at an American Legion meeting in 1976.
Medical microbiologist	A doctor who studies the science of the isolation and identification of micro-organisms that cause diseases in humans and applies this knowledge to treat, control and prevent infections in humans.
Methicillin	A type of antibiotic which used to be used to treat staphylocci infections and is now used in the laboratory as a marker for resistance.
Micro organism	An organism too small to be seen with the naked eye. The term includes bacteria, fungi, protozoa, viruses and some of algae.
Microbiology	The science of the isolation and identified of micro-organisms. Medical microbiology is concerned with those micro-organisms which cause diseases in human.
Microbial pathogen	A micro-organism capable of causing disease.
Morbidity	The state of being diseased, or in a reduced state of health.
Mortality	Death.
MRSA (Methicillin Resistant Staphylococcus aureus)	A strain of Staphylococcus aureus that is resistant to methicillin and has various patterns of other antibiotic resistance.

MSSA (Methicillin Sensitive Staphyloccus aureus)	A strain of Staphylococcus aureus that is sensitive to methicillin.
Multi resistance	A micro-organism that is resistant to two or more unrelated anti-microbial agents.
Mycobacterium tuberculosis	The bacterium which causes tuberculosis (TB).
Negative pressure rooms	The air cycle is controlled so that the pressure inside the room is less than the pressure outside the room thereby ensuring a net inflow of air preventing any micro-organisms passing outside the room.
NICE (National Institute of Clinical Excellence	NICE was set up as a Special Health Authority on 1st April 1999 and as such is part of the NHS. Its role is to provide the NHS with authoritative, robust and reliable guidance on current "best practice". This guidance covers individual health technologies and the clinical management of specific conditions.
Normal flora	The micro-organisms that normally live on or in the body. Also called commensal organisms, they do not cause disease and help to provide protection from infection. When antimicobial agents are used to treat infectious disease they can affect the normal flora and disrupt their ability to provide protection against infection.
Nosocomial	Hospital acquired.
Outbreak	An incident in which two or more people have the same disease, similar symptoms or excrete the same pathogens, and in which there is a time/place/person association. Also a situation where the observed number of cases unaccountably exceeds the expected number.
PHLS (Public Health Laboratory Service	A Government funded organisation of public laboratories based in district, general and teaching hospitals in England and Wales, and a central facility at Colindale in North London which houses the headquarters, National Reference Laboratories and Communicable Disease Surveillance Centre. Its purpose is to protect the population from infection.
Prevalence	The total number of cases of a specific disease in existence in a given population at a certain time.
Prophylaxis	Any means taken to prevent disease. For example, vaccination, or giving antibiotics when patients undergo surgery.

Protective isolation	A type of isolation designed to protect the immuno-compromised patient from infections from other patients, health workers, family, friends and the environment.
Protozoan	A single cell micro-organism that has a true nucleus and a complex and bigger structure than a bacterium. It may be free living or parasitic.
Regional Epidemiologist(s)	A medically qualified consultant specialising in epidemiology and working with a regional unit of the Public Health Laboratory Service Communicable Disease Surveillance Centre.
Regression analysis	A set of statistical techniques the purpose of which is to quantify the relationship between two or more variables.
Resistant micro-organisms	Micro-organisms that are not killed or prevented from replicating by the usual concentrations of an anti-microbial agent.
Screening	Involves taking swabs from patients and staff which are then subject to microbiology testing to determine whether they are colonised or infected by specific micro-organisms eg MRSA.
Sensitive micro-organism	Micro-organisms that are killed or prevented from replicating by the usual concentration of an anti-microbial agent.
Sharps	Items suchs as needles, scalpels etc which can lacerate or puncture the skin.
Source isolation	Aims to prevent the transfer of pathogens or anti-microbial resistant organisms from infected patients to other patients or staff.
Staphylococcus	A group of bacteria which cause a wide variety of infections especially of skin and wounds. More serious infections include blood-poisoning and pneumonia as well as heart valve, bone and joint infections.
Sterilisation	The process by which micro-organisms are destroyed or removed.
Surveillance	Systematic collection of data from the population at risk, identification of infections using consistent definitions, analysis of these data and dissemination of the results to those responsible for the care of the patients and to those responsible for implementation of prevention and control measures.
Toxin	Any poisonous substance produced by a living organism.
Tuberculosis (TB)	An infectious disease most commonly affecting the lungs. Treatment with antibiotics takes many months.

Virus A very small micro-organism of simple structure, only capable of surviving within a living host cell

Appendix 1
Audit methodology

Research methodology

1   We used a variety of techniques to address the study issues set out in Part 1:

- A census of all Acute NHS Trusts and commissioning analyses of responses, including multivariate analysis;

- Audit visits to trusts;

- Review of published literature and attendance at conferences;

- A visit to the Center for Disease Control and Prevention in Atlanta, USA;

- Convening a panel of experts and wider consultation.

The census of all Acute NHS Trusts in England and analysis of results

2   In July 1998, we conducted a census in England of 219 NHS Trusts that provide acute services, based on a self completion postal audit programme. The audit programme was piloted at seven NHS Trusts and was discussed with the NHS Executive and an Expert Panel (see paragraph 14 for details).

3   The audit programme was in two parts: Part 1 was sent to the NHS Trust chief executive to complete and Part 2 was for the infection control team to complete (see Box 1). The programme was designed to test compliance with the Department's guidance and standards, in particular the Department's 1995 guidance on the control of infections in hospitals. This guidance was prepared by the Hospital Infection Working Group of the Department and Public Health Laboratory Service and was issued under HSC (95) 10 as "Department of Health policy". At the time of the census this was the main guidance on the management and control of hospital acquired infection.

Box 1   **Areas covered by the audit programme**

Part 1 - to be completed by NHS Trust Chief Executive

Section A : Details about the NHS Trust

Location, population served, type of NHS Trust, number of admissions, number of beds, type and number of beds in each specialty.

Section B: Infection Control Arrangements

Responsibilities for infection control, including role of the chief executive, extent of coverage of infection control in contracts with health authorities, role of the Trust Board, membership and effectiveness of Hospital Infection Control Committee, infection control guidance and standards used by the Trust.

Part 2 - to be completed by the Infection Control Team

Section A: Infection control policies, guidance and protocols

Existence, contents and review of infection control strategy and annual programmes; and types of policy guidance and protocols used in the Trust and date of last review.

Section B: Infection control activities

Extent and types of surveillance; collection of infection rate data and feedback of results; participation in, and views on, the Nosocomial Infection National Surveillance Scheme (NINSS); extent, types and audit of training and education; monitoring and reporting of hospital hygiene; clinical audit of infection control activity and extent of infection control team's involvement in audits of other clinical and support services (e.g. purchase of new equipment, alterations to hospital buildings); management arrangements for and prevention of out-breaks; extent of staff and patient screening; summary of activities and actual and planned time spent by the infection control doctor and infection control nurse on each compared to the ideal.

Section C: Impact of infection control practices and procedures on hospital acquired infection

Evaluation of infection control measures used in the Trust including any cost benefit analysis these activities; estimates of the level of hospital acquired infection preventable in trusts; participation and impact of accreditation schemes.

Section D: Resources

Numbers and types of infection control doctors and nurses employed; use of and effectiveness of the link nurse system; level and adequacy of clerical support; effectiveness of the Consultant in Communicable Disease Control; level and sources of funds for infection control, availability and content of separate budgets; use of isolation facilities; access to IT support.

4   The census administration, response follow up and data input was conducted by Harris Research; extensive validation checks were carried out on the data provided by Trusts which were "double-entered" to ensure a very high standard of accuracy.

5   In January 1999, we produced the overall quantitative analysis of the completed audit programmes based on 216 full responses out of 219. Further qualitative analyses were completed in February 1999. At the time of finalising the data analysis in April 1999, we had a 100 per cent response rate. Late returns were included in our analysis of open questions, and where relevant, in our evaluation of infection control nurse/bed ratios and infection control doctor/bed ratios (based on how many sessions infection control doctors spent on infection control in their NHS Trusts to the size of the Trust).

6   We attempted to use multivariate analysis to determine whether there were any clear relationships between hospital acquired infection rates and measures designed to prevent and control infections. Relevant variables used were: the amount of funds and time spent on various infection control activities; nurse/bed ratios; whether infection rate data were collected by organism; whether infection rate data were collected by clinical activity; whether infection rate data were collected in some other way; whether infection rates were produced; whether infection trends were produced; and whether the infection control team considered that rates had increased, decreased or stayed the same. A lack of comparable data across a sufficient number of NHS Trusts meant that this proved inconclusive.

The full database of results from the survey was shared with the Department

7   At the time of our census, the Department's regional epidemiologists were planning a similar survey. To avoid duplication and minimise the burden on individual NHS Trusts, we informed Trusts in an advance joint National Audit Office and Department of Health letter, that we would give the Department of Health's regional epidemiologists access to the results of our census. No objections were received from NHS Trusts. The regional epidemiologists analysed our data on a regional and individual Trust basis. They are using the results to work with regional Directors of Public Health to improve the overall management and control of hospital acquired infection. We have provided each participating Trust with a report on our analysis of their own performance on several key areas and how this compares with the national picture. The analysis work to produce the individual NHS Trust reports was carried out by Nergish Desai, Academic Assistant, Department of Medical Microbiology, King's College London.

Audit visits and wider consultations

8   Detailed audit visits were carried out during the pilot and full stage to obtain further information, follow up examples of good practice, and test our audit findings. We visited:

- Chase Farm Hospital NHS Trust

- Colchester General Hospital NHS Trust

- Crawley Hospital NHS Trust

- Royal Surrey County Hospital NHS Trust (Guildford)

- Stoke Mandeville NHS Hospital Trust

- University College London NHS Hospital Trust

- King's Healthcare NHS Trust

- St George's Healthcare NHS Trust

- Frimley Park Hospitals NHS Trust

- North Manchester Healthcare NHS Trust

- Central Nottinghamshire Health Care NHS Trust

- Trent Health Authority

- Manchester Health Authority

- Homerton Hospital NHS Trust

- The Nosocomial Infection National Surveillance Unit

- The Public Health Laboratory Service

- The London School of Hygiene and Tropical Medicine

9   We consulted with Royal Colleges (Surgeons, Pathologists, Nursing, Paediatrics and Child Health, Orthopaedics, Anaesthetists, General Practitioners, Obstetrics and Gynaecology), the Health and Safety Executive, Infection Control Nurses Association, Hospital Infection Society, United Kingdom Central Council for Nurses, British Medical Association and the National Association of Theatre Nurses, the House of Lords Science and Technology Select Committee and the House of Commons Health Select Committee.

Reliance on the work of other bodies

10   At the outset of the National Audit Office investigation the Department of Health agreed that we could use the results of a costing study by the Central Public Health Laboratory and the London School of Hygiene and Tropical Medicine - The Socio Economic Burden of Hospital Acquired Infection. This was commissioned by the Department to give them some much needed information on the cost of hospital acquired infection. Their report was published on 18 January 2000. At the same time the Nosocomial Infection National Surveillance Scheme team at the Public Health Laboratory Service agreed to share with us the results of the first full years national data on hospital acquired bacteraemias surgical site infections. The report on surgical site infection was published in December 1999, and a report on the first two years on bacteraemias results is expected to be published soon.

Review of published literature and attendance at conferences

11   We carried out literature searches and extensive reviews of published literature on the extent and cost of hospital acquired infection and good practice relating to various infection control activities, including infection control arrangements in other European countries and in the USA. We also drew on the evidence presented to the House of Lords Select Committee on Science and Technology and their 1998 Report on Resistance to Antibiotics and other Microbial Agents and the Government's response to this, and on a paper presented by the Department to the House of Commons Health Select Committee.

12   We attended a number of workshops and conferences. The main conferences attended were: the 4th International Conference of the Hospital Infection Society, September 1998; the 28th Annual Infection Control Nurses Association Conference, September 1998; and the 29th Annual Infection Control Nurses Association Conference, September 1999.

22 Regional Services Division, Public Health Laboratory Service Communicable Disease Surveillance Centre (1997). A Survey of the Communicable Disease Control Function in England. London: Public Health Laboratory Service.

23 Crawshaw S, Roberts J, Allen P, Taylor L, Croxson B (1999). Risks and infectious diseases in managed markets. Economic and Social Research Council, *Grant Number* L21130200438.

24 House of Lords Select Committee on Science and Technology (1998). Resistance to Antibiotics –Evidence. London: Stationery Office.

25 Royal College of Pathologists (1999). Medical and Scientific Staffing of NHS Pathology Departments. London: Royal College of Pathologists.

26 Department of Health (1998). Information for Health – An Information Strategy for the Modern NHS, HSC/168. London: Department of Health.

27 Gaynes RP, Solomon S (1996). Improving hospital acquired infection rates: The CDC Experience. *Journal on Quality Improvement* 22: No7, 457-467

28 The Advisory Group on Infection, Scottish Office (1998). Scottish Infection Control Manual. Scottish Office.

29 Gould D J (1995). Hand decontamination: nurses opinions and practices *Nursing Times* 91: (17): 42-5.

30 Gould D J, Wilson-Barnett J (1996). Nurses infection control practices. *International Journal of Nursing Studies* 33:143-160.

31 Teare E L, Cookson B, French G, Gould D, Jenner E, McCulloch J, Pallett A, Scwieger M, Scott G, Wilson J (1999) Handwashing. A modest measure with big effects. *British Medical Journal* 318 page 686.

32 Handwashing Liaison Group - Hospital Infection Society/Association of Medical Microbiologists/Department of Health/Infection Control Nurses Association /Royal College of Nursing /Public Health Laboratory Service (1999). Hospital Acquired Infection: Information for Chief Executives - Why *you* need to be interested! Sent to Chief Executives of NHS Trusts by the Department of Health - March 1999.

33 Hampshall P, Thomson M (1998). Grime Watch. *Nursing Times* 16(94) 37: 66-69.

34 Wilcox M H, Cunniffee J G, Trundel, Redpath (1996). Financial burden of hospital acquired *Clostridium difficile* infection. *Journal of Hospital Infection* 34: 23-30.

35 Ludlam H, Brown N, Sule O, Redpath C, Cori N, Owen G (1990) An antibiotic policy is associated with reduced risk of *Clostridium difficile* – associated diarrhoea. *Age and Ageing* 28-6.

36 Millward S, Barnett J, Thomlinson D (1993). Clinical infection control audit programme evaluation of an audit tool that is used by infection control nurses to monitor standards and assess effective staff training. *Journal Hospital Infection* 24: 219-232.

Reports by the Comptroller and Auditor General, Session 1999-2000

The Comptroller and Auditor General has to date, in Session 1999-2000, presented to the House of Commons the following reports under Section 9 of the National Audit Act, 1983:

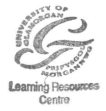

Learning Resources
Centre

Printed in the UK for The Stationery Office on behalf of the
Controller of Her Majesty's Stationery Office
Dd.5067452, 2/00, 5673, Job No.TJ 000556

The Management and Control of Hospital Acquired Infection in Acute NHS Trusts in England

Ordered by the
House of Commons
to be printed 14 February 2000

LONDON: The Stationery Office
£14.20

HC 230 Session 1999–00
Published 17 February 2000

This report has been prepared under Section 6 of the National Audit Act 1983 for presentation to the House of Commons in accordance with Section 9 of the Act.

John Bourn
Comptroller and Auditor General

National Audit Office
7 February 2000

1189329 X

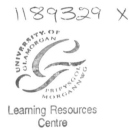

Learning Resources
Centre

The Comptroller and Auditor General is the head of the National Audit Office employing some 750 staff. He, and the National Audit Office, are totally independent of Government. He certifies the accounts of all Government departments and a wide range of other public sector bodies; and he has statutory authority to report to Parliament on the economy, efficiency and effectiveness with which departments and other bodies have used their resources.

For further information about the National Audit Office please contact:

National Audit Office
Press Office
157-197 Buckingham Palace Road
Victoria
London
SW1W 9SP

Tel: 0171-798 7400

email:nao@gtnet.gov.uk

Web site address: http://www.nao.gov.uk